3 Trimesters_ For Life

Compiled By...

Heart's Database & Team

Copyright © 2020 by **FAMIAN**

All rights reserved.
"3 Trimesters for Life"
ISBN: 978-1-71695-654-6

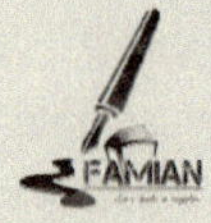

Published by **FAMIAN**

Email:
famian.onl9@gmail.com

DISCLAIMER

*This book is a collection of real stories.
Names, characters, places, and incidents either are the
product of the author's real life or are used with the
permission of actual person.*

CATALOGING-IN-PUBLICATION DATA

Title:	3 Trimesters for Life
Author Type:	Multiple
Book Type:	Stories & Quotes
Genre:	Self Help/Motherhood
Self Published by:	**FAMIAN**
Concept by:	Kamlesh Mishra and Syed Faiz Ibrahim
Cover Design by:	Syed Faiz Ibrahim and Nikita Yadav
Content Support By:	Lalitha Priyadharshini and Gayatri Barnwal
Edited by:	Aman Sharma and Syed Faiz Ibrahim
Proof Read by:	Ritika Soni, Kinjal Khanna and Panchanand Gupta
Document Designing and Marketing Support by:	Keval Suchak and Nikita Yadav

OUR ASSOCIATIVE PLATFORMS

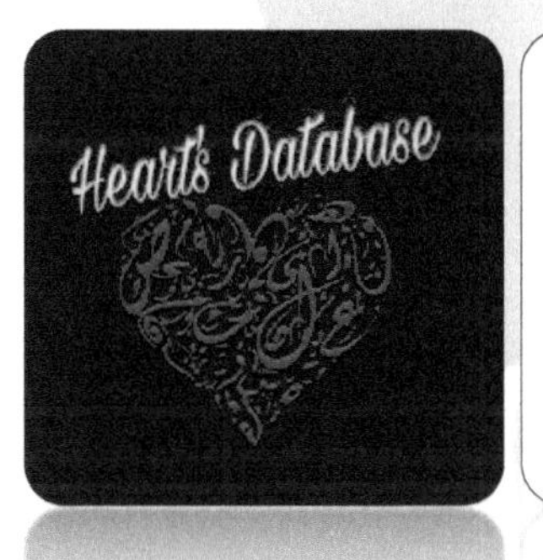

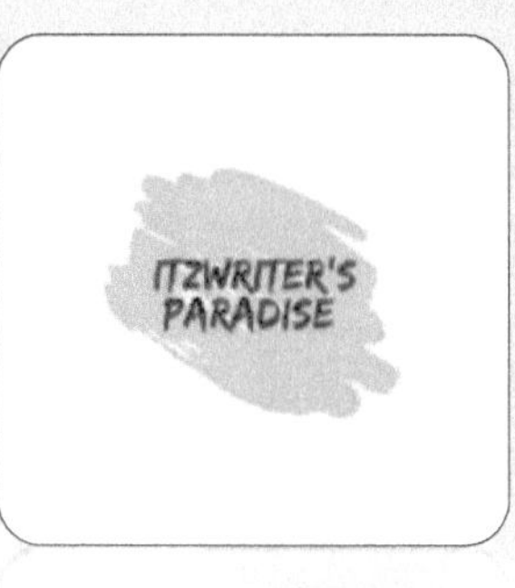

Special Thanks To...

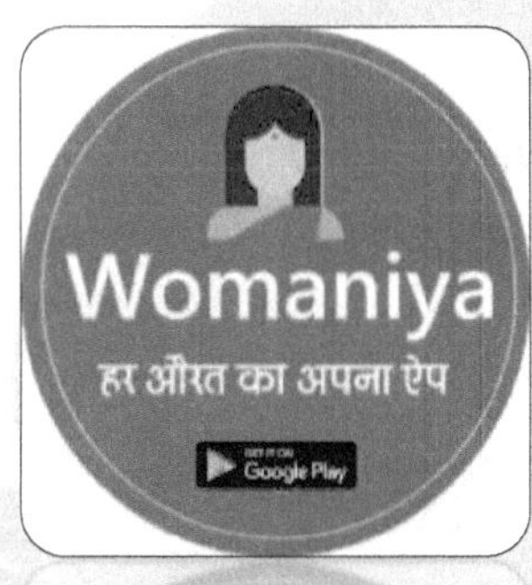

OUR SPONSORS...

Institute Sponsors...

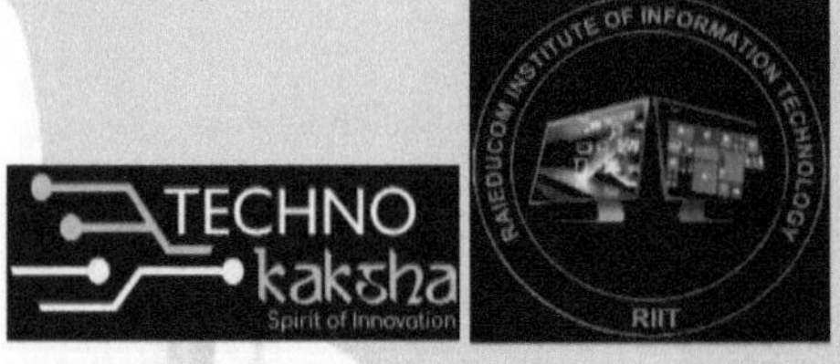

Literary Sponsors...

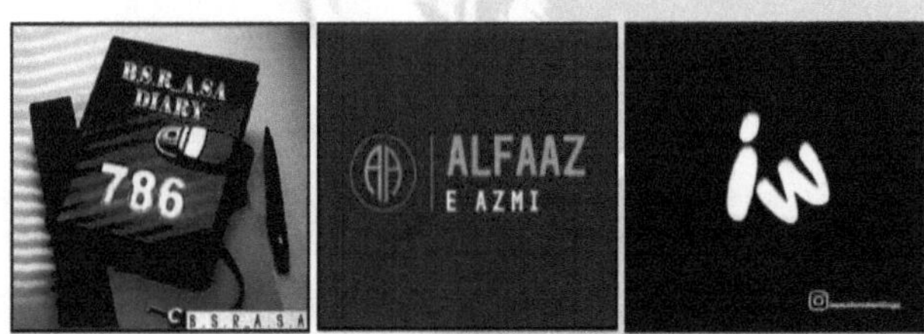

Corporate Sponsors...

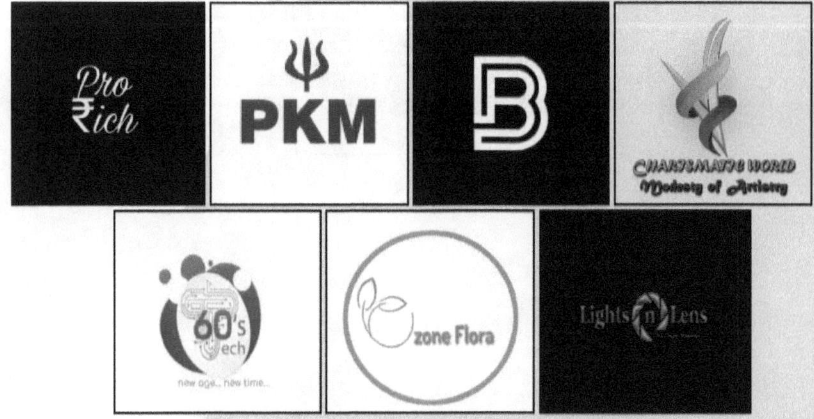

Dedicated to all mothers out there for their unconditional love in the universe

ACKNOWLEDGEMENT

First and foremost, praises and thanks to the God, the Almighty, for his showers of blessings throughout the course of our work for this book.

We express our gratitude to each and every author associated with this book. A special thanks to **Womaniya** app for connecting with us. We also express our sincere gratitude to our institute sponsors-**Techno Kaksha** and **Raieducom Institute of Information Technology(RIIT)**, our literary sponsors- **B.S.R A.S.A Diary 786, Alfaaz-e-Azmi** and **Immatured Writings,**our corporate sponsors- **Pro Rich, PK Metals, Charismatic World, Tech 60's, Brandit, Ozone Flora** and **LightnLens** for their valuable contribution.

We are indebted to **Priyal Vasoya, Chetna Bhatia** and **Shamim Merchant** who were always there whenever we needed any help. A Special thanks to each of our FAMIAN team members for their constant and time-to-time support. Last but not the least, a big thanks to our whole team of "3 Trimesters for Life." Without them and their co-operation, completion of this book would have been inevitable and their presence behind us was totally indispensable.

CONTENTS

INTRODUCTION

Every person has their own meaning to life. Creation of life is so pure. Trimesters in a women's life is the time when God gifts her power of creation. We have seen so many love stories in literature but no love can take a stand in front of mother's love for her child. The time when woman starts feeling happy instead of anxious due to the growing stomach, is when she realizes that she has to take care of herself but not for herself. Pregnancy is when she sees her beauty, not due to perfect shape but due to love developing inside her. Those trimesters, she's not only carrying the baby but she loves and protects her child with her life.

The journey of physical, hormonal and emotional alteration along with doubting habit is a roller coaster ride. She knows all about the pain that she have to bear during child birth yet she only smiles with happiness thinking about that time. It's a pure bliss for her to bring her child into the world. The three trimesters of life is a spectrum of emotions. The fascinating feeling of tiny movements in the womb reminds her that she is never alone. The three trimesters makes her realize how strong she is. It gives rise to qualities of godliness to a woman.

There are many beauties of pregnancy, how looking at tiny clothes melts the heart, how ladies plan to decorate the baby room, how difficult it is to sleep with round belly but in same time, she feels her baby is sleeping inside her, how ladies crave for food in this time. At the same time, there are many hustling anxious thoughts and painful moments too. Babies bring a new meaning to her life and she would see the world in a different eyes. Trimesters are not a period to bring child into the world but the period filled with love and happiness.

What do you think, a mom will ask if God gifts her a wish? Obviously, without any doubt she would use that single wish for her children. That is the difference between mom and any other relationship; mom would sacrifice anything to protect her child. That's how special mom is.

Every mother has a unique story that can't be explained in just few words, so Trimesters is designed where you can read about happy and painful stories of motherhood. You can know how the beauty of motherhood fills colours of happiness in the life of a woman.

Divine Journey

~*Masuma Oomatia*

otherhood is a dream of every woman. It is a priceless gift of nature to a woman. After one and a half years of our marriage, my husband and I decided to begin a family. Both of us are from medical backgrounds, so, we were aware of ovulation cycles and planned accordingly . I wanted my child to be born before the month of June so my child should not lose time in school admission.

By the grace of God, I conceived soon. When I missed my periods, I was very excited but we both were cautious as sometimes your strong desire and imaginations can also have an impact on menstrual cycle.

After six weeks, my pregnancy test showed positive results. I still remember my first morning sickness timing. We went to see our family friends. At their house, their children were having afternoon tea. I had a strong desire to eat bread with margarine. It was Blue band margarine. I still recollect the taste of it. I loved it, but immediately I felt sick and I could not hold it. I rushed to her kitchen sink. My friend merrily looked at me. I still remembers happiness on her face.

Throughout my pregnancy, I kept on vomiting. I used to throw everything out soon after eating. Sometimes vomiting was so violent that I used to pass out for a few seconds. But every time after this 'sickness' I used to thank God that he gave me an opportunity to conceive. Feeling of having a new life in your body was an amazing experience. There are no words to express it.

First 3 months passed with exhausting morning sickness, I couldn't bear the smell of food and I used to ask my husband to join me in the kitchen so that talking would divert my mind. My husband was very supportive. I was vomiting 3-4 times a day; he encouraged me to eat healthy food.

Generally, Indian women are anaemic. My husband made sure that I ate an egg regularly for good iron intake. Along with it, he used to give me orange juice so, in the presence of vitamin C, iron absorption is good.

We informed both our family and all were happy.

My first ultrasound...Oh my God! I could see a small hand. I cried in gratitude. Ultrasound operator asked me if I wanted to know the sex of my baby. I said,"NO!". I was happy to accept whatever God gave me. However I wanted to have a girl. Expected delivery date of my baby was 7th May.

The most awaited date of my life.

In my second semester of pregnancy, vomiting continued along with headaches. Now began the monthly routine checkup with the midwife. My weight was increasing exponentially.In the middle of the fifth month, one day while cooking, I felt a thud in my abdomen. It was the first kick of my baby. I felt many kicks that afternoon. I was thrilled and was eagerly waiting to share this wonderful experience with my husband. In the evening when he came I took his hand and put it on my abdomen. But - no luck. We waited the whole evening but my poor husband did not have any joy. He went to sleep. I was awake with happiness. My baby started moving again. Now it had become a routine, my baby was more active at night. I was getting rolly-polly. My abdomen started showing a good sized bump. Six months passed without any mishap. Thank God.

In my third semester, vomiting continued with headaches and now there were more sleepless nights. I started getting heartburn as well; I had to avoid all types of spicy food. But our enthusiasm was building up. Only a few more months and our baby would be in our arms.

I started visiting baby stores. Started enjoying looking at the baby clothes and all the accessories, new born baby needs. We both were enjoying our window shopping. It was very hard to control our temptation to buy things for our first child. My mother came to support me in April, just a month before. I was more relaxed and started enjoying mummy's handmade food. As she knew how to make delicious food without chillies and spices. I was getting bigger and bigger. Difficult to lie down. I was counting days.

On 1st May my mother and I were relaxing, listening to a spiritual audio. One side of the cassette finished, to change the side I got up from bed. I had a severe abdominal spasm. I screamed. My mum tried to put me at ease, suggesting maybe labor pains had started, as we were only a week away from EDD. I was shocked.

To recover from my anxiety, my mum helped me divert my mind, she suggested that let's get ready in case we need to go to hospital tonight. I occupied myself. No more spasms. I thanked the lord for postponing my delivery date. Whole night passed peacefully. My husband assured me that it is normal to get occasional spasms. Maybe it was due to awkward postures. My EDD passed, nothing happened.

On 9th May, I went to see my doctor. He examined me. He looked worried; he couldn't locate the baby's head. Immediately he sent me for an ultrasound. All were shocked. My baby had turned 180°. Doctor told my husband, " Your wife is 5 feet tall and carrying a big baby as a 6 feet tall mother would carry. Your baby is intelligent, last minute changed the position. Now due to breech position, normal delivery will be difficult. We have to get your baby out by cesarean section." I was shocked and very upset that I will not be able to give birth to my baby normally. I was now full term. We had to give consent for the surgery.

11th May, when I recovered from anesthesia, my husband brought my beautiful son to me. I couldn't believe that he was my baby. Beautiful round pinkish face, dark thick black hair, big eyes, dark long eyelashes. God's "ASIM" blessing showered upon us. "ASIM," my son, his name means limitless. Tears were rolling down my face. My husband hugged me. All the pain and exhaustion of the last 3 trimesters simply vanished. We both were grateful and felt complete.

*****

*"Life doesn't come with a bed full of roses.
It comes with a mother who's love is
eternal for the rest of her life"*

~Rishav Banerjee

Life Beyond Us

~Shamim Merchant

Motherhood, the most prestigious designation in spite of all hardships. Filled with nostalgic memories, here are reminiscences of the birth of my first son.

Marriage happened at a very young age of 22. Within three months into the nuptials, I had conceived and was expecting my first child. Although it was an amazing feeling, I wanted some quality time with my husband before beginning a family. Nevertheless, my gynaecologist said that it was the right age for motherhood. Congratulations poured in and everyone was elated. Now began my painful journey of pregnancy. My doctor aunt guided me at each step, regarding my daily routine and diet. I read a lot and saw videos too. But truth be told, in such circumstances, you don't gain much from another's experience. Every woman's trimester is unique and each one has a special story to tell.

Hormonal changes started showing its colours and I was nauseatic for most part of the days. My 'Good morning' began with vomiting. I cooked with a handkerchief over my nose and couldn't bear the smell of food. I landed up not eating anything I made. I survived only on fruits and juices. My gynaecologist pacified me that these symptoms would defuse within a couple of months. Hardly! I vomited all nine months. Believe me; I couldn't tolerate my husband's intimacy. Even that triggered nausea. I was a very thin girl and my waist was merely 24 inches. But my baby belly changed all that. As months progressed and took me deeper into pregnancy, at full term, the circumference of my waist was 59 inches. It shocks me even today; I had actually stretched to that extent.

As trimesters unfolded further, vomiting became a routine and I got used to it. Now the major issue was blood pressure. It runs in hereditary. My husband, doctor and me, we were all worried about it. My BP constantly remained high, around 250. A lot of diet control was advised. Obviously, medicines had to be avoided. We didn't want to put my baby through any danger. I had to stop going for walks. My legs suffered permanent swelling and I had to sit and sleep with legs raised high. Cushions became my best friends and I was practically never without them. My wardrobe had a complete makeover and my mirror reflected a totally different person. I loved the brand new me and was proud of my baby-bump. Previously, I had learnt tailoring and knitting. It came in handy and I happily made lots of colourful, soft tiny clothes for my little bundle of joy. Though I didn't know the sex of the child, but still. Motherly feelings are always at a different level.

We live in Mumbai and during my seventh month, my mom took me to Bangalore. I was going to deliver there. In Bangalore, my first visit to the hospital saw more check-ups, concerns, advices and prescribed supplements. I became heavier with each passing day and found it difficult to carry myself. My baby-bump was so large that when standing, I couldn't see my own feet. Swollen feet compelled me to wear flats bigger than my usual size.

26th August 1993, was the given due date. Nonetheless, high BP and sleeping with raised feet, showed no signs of my baby moving down. On the 'The Day', at eleven in the morning, my amniotic sac bursted. Since weeks, my hospital bag was ready, positioned near the main door. Mom called up dad and asked him to meet us at the hospital. I pinged my aunt. She assured to be by my side till the end. When I rang up Iqbal, my husband, he wished me luck and expressed his love and affection for both of us. I promised to keep him updated. Mobiles weren't invented then and for some reason, he couldn't be with us.

After the required check-ups, my gynaecologist smiled, "You've wisely come at the right time." She hollered for a nurse, asked her to put me on a wheelchair and guided me to the labor room. I was strictly prohibited from walking after that. The hospital was humongous and the gynaec ward was nearly 1000 meters away. I still had no signs of contractions.

It's a blessing to have a sympathetic staff at the clinic. They don't reduce the pain, but certainly make it bearable. After my bathroom rituals, I was put on the delivery gurney. An IV was fixed and pain inducing meds were injected in the bottle. Mom was told to wait outside. I was freaking hysterical, nothing less than a bundle of jittery nerves. Completely panic stricken. But praise the lord, my aunt was allowed to be by my side. Slowly and steadily I sensed the first indication of labor pains. Gradually they increased in frequency and force, to the point of being devastatingly intolerable. It was the most exaggerated time of my life. Childbirth saw the extreme of everything in me. My deepest prayers, my puffed up short breaths and my loudest screams. All along I held a death grip on my aunt's hand. I knew my hold was bruising her limb, but I was helpless.

My aunt and my doctor patiently kept pouring words of encouragement in my ears. Needless to say, they meant nothing to me at that time. I was fighting for life and wasn't sure if I would come out alive from all this. After six hours of agonizing pain, my gynaec could only see the head of my baby. He was a big boy. She had to use forceps to help him slip out.

My world, my baby boy, all soaked up in mix fluids was in my doctor's hands and just like that, all the pain and complains against the universe, disappeared in a fraction of a second. An amalgam of tears and smiles enveloped my face. In that moment, I wanted nothing else but to hold my baby in my arms. God had truly showered his choicest blessings on me in the form of my beautiful angel, my boy- 'Shams'. His name means 'The Sun'. He was given in my arms and I immediately fed him. The nostalgic moment cannot be described in words. My heart was dancing in my chest, overflowing with joy and thankfulness. My smiles and my tears, were unstoppable. I was missing my husband profusely. We badly needed a threesome hug.

He's a miracle, a child from heaven on earth,
No one can ever measure his worth.
He's unique and special – my little dove,
A beautiful souvenir of our united love.

*****

> *"Mothers are the most courageous creations in the cosmos who endure pain with pleasurable face"*
>
> *~Gayathri Rithyaga*

Colors Of Smile

~Durga Bhavani

Being a mother is a very good news that woman hears for her complete life. A bit of fear, a bit of tension,the more excitement, that more and more happiness which can't be gained again and again. The nine months, three trimesters, 39 to 40 weeks, approximately 280 days.

There was a baby, who was growing day by day, in my womb. Shared with me, lived with me! Nausea, mood swings and morning sickness was common at the first stage.

The care shown by the family and my husband really made me feel something special. I used to have monthly check ups. All the time my husband couldn't be my side because of his office works. Yet I was not alone; my baby gave me all time company no matter where I go.

It was about to reach seventh month, the gynaecologist said that the baby in my womb was in reverse position and deliver might be critical! So I used to have a morning walks for almost two hours.

The days passed on and the delivery time arrived.

My husband was not by my side, some of my relatives suggested me the government hospital and said that they also treat well. They admitted me in the government hospital which is in a village.

I felt the pain of hell. No healing words from my husband as he was not there beside me. I was suffering with the pains. There was no doctor in the hospital. And I wished the

Almighty "just for once let me see my baby" as I thought I can't stay alive for the long time. After sometime one of the nurses decided to operate me.

Slowly I got relief from the labor pains. I was not conscious. But I heard the words said by nurse to the other one "as we are late, the living chances of both might be hard". And now I just wished to keep my baby alive. But luckily we both are safe. I heard the cry of my baby in the operation theater.

None of the mother can forget the first cry of their babies, the first kiss to those tiny lips and hands.

*****

"When she hears your cry for the first time she forgets all her pain and tries to lean over to look at your face and smile"

~Dinesh Bissa

Unexpected Blessing

~Chetna Bhatia

onth of June brought me the news of being pregnant ,after 7 months of my marriage. I accepted it with mixed feelings. I did not know whether to be happy or worried as our financial condition was very bad.

Family was facing a huge loss in business. The news did not bring much of joy to the family as it should have been for the 'first grandchild' of the family.

At the young age of 23, in the era of - Rajeshri productions - Salman khan movies like *'Hum aapke hai kaun'*, I too dreamt of those cozy and happy moments when the news was be announced to husband and family. 'Ahh!!! .... It just happens in the movie. Maybe not in real world.'

Anyways, I was taken to the doctor to ask if it could be aborted. I just walked along like a Zombie. Age of 23 was too young to think of all this, react or go against the family decision. The doctor was strictly against it. Her words brought back life in me. I wanted to feel that happiness, that special feeling, that joy.....

I looked around but there was no one to join me. Days passed, the happiest was my husband and my brother-in- law. A cute gesture I still remember, he had brought a packet of almonds and said *"Bhabhi Roj Khana"*. That was so touching. I will never ever forget that buying almonds during that bad financial condition was a big thing.

I could feel changes in my body as the months passed. Now slowly I had started telling myself, "I have another life inside me. I have to take care of it more than myself". I used to read spiritual books. I used to go for the regular checkups to the best Gynaecologist. She was a family friend.

Everything was fine, the only change I felt through my pregnancy was I used to feel very lethargic by afternoon, I felt like resting or taking a nap but the comments from the neighbouring aunty scared the family members *"Dopahar ko Soyegi toh ladki hi Aaegi."*

What the hell?"

I used to feel, "How does it matter whether it's a girl or a boy or how does the sleep connect with the gender of the baby?"

Two trimesters were over. We had a small function for *'Gaud bharai'.* That was the first time my parents visited my home. I was very happy as I was meeting them after a very long time. One day, I had some guest at home and as usual and as a good daughter in law, I had to be a good host to them. Special mention here, I live on the fourth floor with no lift. By late evening, I felt a little worked up as I had gone down 6 to 7 times to bring the required things. After finishing my chores, at around 11:00 p.m, I laid down on my bed feeling exhausted. Suddenly, I felt the flow of water. I got scared and I did not know what to do. I told my husband and in-laws' about it.

We rushed to the hospital. It was Christmas Eve, the doctor was about to leave for the party. She gave me an injection and asked me to get admitted and left. Though the flow of water had reduced, it continued through the night and in few hours I was in severe pain. Early morning around 5.00 the doctor was called. On checking she said the condition was critical and the delivery has to happen at that very moment. I was shocked. The due date was in February. It was seventh month. I had also heard survival chances of seventh month babies are very rare. It was very risky. She also said she will try her best but does not promise anything.

While entering the operation theatre, I remembered the words of the people they use to say "I was so lucky that I did not have any problem throughout my pregnancy".

At that time, for a minute my heart said, *"Nazar Lag gai Sabki."*

In next 20 minutes, a baby girl was born who was very weak, only 1.8 kg and she turned blue. I was still unconscious. Being a premature baby, she was to be kept in that incubator in some other Hospital.

After sometime, my husband came in, hugged me tight and broke down while repeating the doctor's words, "The baby is to be considered to be yours only when we hand over to you. We will try our best but chances are very less."

First time l saw a strong man in tears. That time l felt it's not a man who is crying but a father. I turned into a statue. I still get jitters when I remember those moments.

My baby was handed over to me after 45 days. That was the day I got my new life. By God's grace, she was hail and healthy ever after. But till date whenever that episode runs through my mind, I breakdown.

*****

*"The stretch marks on her tummy tells
the story of forty weeks of her journey
and the wait to embrace her child"*

~Kayathri Kumar

Platform Of Delight

~Sushama Pahade

I am feeling very happy to share my story with you. One needs to take many efforts to become mature because the special feeling of becoming a mother is understood by only a woman. My story is not special but it is a gift for me from God.

When I was 21, I got married. Due to big family, I not only became mature but also responsible. I spent my 1st year by taking care of others. After some months, I started feeling dizzy. My husband was in the government hospital, so I used to take medicine at my home. I thought maybe it was happening due to much work I was doing and hence, I went for the check-up. We were getting the report at evening.

My husband said, "Don't worry; I will bring your report at evening while coming from office. You just take care."

After coming home, he sat near me. I was in tension that what actually has happened. But then,that special time came to me when I come to know that "I am becoming a mother". It was a special day because it was for the first time that my husband told me this news. That day was 3rd March 1997, my husband's birthday. When I heard, tears came out of my eyes. Those tears were not of sadness but of the happiness. I was out of control. I didn't know what to do.

As I heard off this good news, I started thinking what to do for the baby. In this way, 3 months passed. Work load increased. I was the only one to work at home and other 5 members were on job. Due to much work, I used to eat 2 times a day or sometimes even 1 time a day. This was my daily routine. I stopped taking any medicine. Whenever I was tired, I used to start thinking about my baby and that thought used to give a new power to work faster. Whenever any festival was there, I used to clean our house along with the utensils and clothes. As there was the problem of water, I used to bring water from well which was far from home.

Nowadays, women do sonography. But at my times, due to poor condition, I decided not to do the sonography. But, I used to imagine my baby and started to live happy. I thought, it's okay if I can't see him/her but I can imagine. 2 months passed by thinking of the baby. The days were passing like normal days but something was special in those days which were making me more excited. Now, I started feeling like baby was growing and I crossed my 6th month.

In 7th month, I was excited for my baby shower. I was thinking about the program that what would happen in the program, which items would be there, what would I select.

After some days, baby shower came. A small but excited program was arranged for me. Relatives, neighbours were called. My mom bought new sari for me. Garland was made of rose and marigold flowers for the waist. All the ladies were singing song to welcome my baby. Some songs were funny and some were spreading more happiness. At last the 'hidden item' game was there for me in which I needed to select a single item which would determine whether it will a girl or a boy.

For example, if one selects *pedha* or *balushai* then it will be a boy and if one selects *jalebi* or *barfi* then it will be a girl. I chose a bowl and I found it was *jalebi*. I was very happy that I would be blessed with a baby girl as Diwali was there in next month. It is said that the girl is born at that house which has destiny. I was having that destiny.

7th month passed and I could feel the baby kicking. My legs were swelling. In spite of feeling tired, I continued with my work and passed my days. I went for the final check-up at hospital to check baby's weight.

Doctor said, "Don't worry, Everything is fine." and I was happy that in spite of being busy, I took good care of baby.

Finally, the day came when I was admitted to hospital at Akola. Due to more weight, it was not possible to do normal delivery and hence doctor decided to do ceaser. She told me to move here and there so that it would be easy for the delivery. Now it was the time for my delivery. They took me to the operation theatre at evening 7:45 and gave anaesthesia.

On 30 November 1997, my baby saw the world. When I was awake, they kept my baby near me. There is only one day in this world when mother smiles on her baby's cry. I just kissed her on forehead because she was the first baby girl after 1 generation.

She was looking so fragile and cute that name came out from my mouth as **"Prajakta"**. It means 'flower'. Everybody liked the name and started calling her as Prajakta.

It is said that the parents are lucky who are blessed with a baby girl. Boy is the Diva of the house but the girl is the light of the house which lightens her family name everywhere and we are lucky to have a daughter.

"The best fighter is a daughter."

*****

"She offers her child with an unconquerable chest, not prone to diseases or calamities for three trimesters, and desires to do the same for three decades"

~Geethanjali Athi

Ceaseless Memory

~*Seetha Lakshmi*

I was brought up in a house of five kids. Being the eldest, my childhood was occupied with itself on growing my younger ones; motherhood has developed in me in my early childhood just because of my siblings. But have always wondered about giving birth.

First Trimester:

It was one fine evening after my marriage, I felt dizzy when I was busy into household chores, thought it's because of too much of works I am engaged into, than usual. I sat down to rest a while. Then, in minutes or two I felt nauseating; As I am alone in home, my husband being off to work, faced the discomfort without sharing to anyone and it was a period when mobile is a wonder. Took a nap in tired. After waking up, I realised I am getting a delay in my periods. In the evening, after my husband's arrival, I explained all those I undergone clearly. He took me to a clinic nearby and I had a check-up.

I found I was pregnant with my first baby, I was literally on cloud nine, have confirmed with doctor and informed about my pregnancy to all my family members, I was asked not to talk about this pregnancy to anyone till I start with my fifth month. I attended all my check-ups without skipping the date given, every time during my check-up, I will be asking 'n' number of questions with doctor regarding the baby's health. The doctor will be saying with smile in her face "baby's growth is too good", it was the only word that used to console my soul.

Since I was a biology student in my school, I knew that my little one is getting all the vital organs developed, so I began eating good food as it should be sufficient for two souls. I began continuing healthy food habits more than before. I used to walk very carefully. Every time I slept, I was very keen on my stomach as the little one was inside me, making sure I don't hurt my little one.

Second Trimester:

My conscience said it should be baby girl. I experienced nausea every time I ate and felt very hard in in-taking food and was feeling dizzy too, only food that I found better was tender coconut and curd rice ; I won't be vomiting only if I had them. My mom and dad visited my place once in two weeks. They wanted me to be with them in my hometown, for my delivery after having baby shower, but my husband denied to send me and promised them that he will care me more than my parents; every time they leave my place I shed tears like a kid, making my husband to care me.

The baby usually twists and turns inside me as if it was a snake or something. I even wonder at times as if it's baby or what and why does this happen, the baby was that much hyper. I used to have an evening walk to the nearest beach daily, will talk for hours with the little one inside me about everything, used to see especially the little girls on the beach road who rides cycle with pony hair every day. As usual I would lost myself into your dreams as a baby girl, when the baby is born, grow up and more other stuffs. I thought too much on raising the little one with high values and morals.

Third Trimester:

It was the most awaited period in my life. I began to get ready for my new one's arrival. My weight got increased than before but doctors said my BMI for pregnancy was normal, making me not to worry about delivery complications. I began getting tired. I felt the baby-bump so perfectly now, than before. Every time I felt the bump, I would dreamt about "Arjuna teaching *Chakra Vyuh* to his son ABIMANYU when he was in his mom's womb", deep down I felt that effect works, so I talked more of good and positive things to the little one inside me always, every day I gave special time for the little one growing inside me. Sometimes I smile at myself for being so childishly matured.

Those days I felt myself proud and I wanted the one inside me too to be very proud for every little thing the little one deserves.

Labor pain began and I was rushed to the hospital, I felt like it was the heaviest of all pain I have to bear in my life, it was on January 1 exactly, the pain prolonged actually for the next day too, doctors began speaking about operating, I didn't want to get operated and asked them if I could wait for the next day too for the baby to come out, they checked my health and gave hope to wait for one more day.

Finally the day came, it was a hour of severe pain all over my abdomen especially in my hip bones, I never cared anything except having the little one out from me safe, the last sound I heard before getting fainted was my little one crying aloud, "Yes, the baby saw the outside world finally and it's a baby girl." My proud little baby girl.

*****

*"A mother is the only person on earth who
can divide the love among her several
children and each child will
have the equal share"*

~Riyanshi Gupta

Heavenly Scars

~Shakun Devi

It was much like any other day. Waking up, getting freshened up, cooking, worshiping, washing dishes and clothes, soiling and cleaning the house, etc and facing my husband, Karan's anger. My mother-in-law never forgets, even for a single day, to curse me. I had served this lady and the family for about 25 years but they never loved me. My son has always been busy studying, as he also wanted to get rid of his father by taking a job. My daughter, Soni used to help me with some errands. Everyone remained busy for almost all the time. Yes, I had not got a good family. Karan was an arrogant, dominating and short tempered husband. There were always quarrels and fights between us. I used to get tired not because of loads of work but because of mental pressure I was made to face in this house. Life had not brought even a small token of happiness for me since a long time.

It was a pleasant morning of 2000. Generally, my husband used to come home with fear for all but that day, he came with a good news,

"We are shifting to our new house", he screamed.

"Really?", I asked.

"Yes, it is near to the railway station where I work." he explained.

"That's good news," Soni said.

We got shifted there in some days. This new place brought another news for me. What people calls as good news was a weird news for me at that time. I started having headaches, weakness and weird kind of feelings. I thought it to be another sign of getting older but after checkup, I came to know that I was pregnant with my fourth child at an age of 40. My third child was 18 years old by then. At first, I hesitated saying this to anyone but I gathered courage to tell my family about this. They looked at me with brows up, but then consoled me by saying, "It's ok." We will have a little angel in our home." Some part of me was happy but some part of me was tensed too. When my stomach started growing, I even stopped attending family functions, going outside and sharing this news with anyone. Some of my neighbours discouraged me from having baby so late.

"Your body in this age is very weak to handle such pain.", someone said.

Some said," Baby born to old moms are very weak".

Someone even mocked, "She is so fond of romance, that she got pregnant at this age."

All these used to scare me alot. I started feeling very awkward to tell anyone. I actually started disliking my pregnancy and the baby because of all this.

Pregnancies are meant to be difficult but it is much more difficult in a conservative family where very little cooperation from the family is expected. All day busy with household works and then the awkward feelings at night used to kill me. It continued for first two months. In those days, I used to love reading newspapers. Fortunate was that pleasant afternoon to present me with an amazing news. It was about the wife of a famous government officer who got pregnant in her 40s. I was really glad and relaxed after reading it. It felt like a burden just got released from my head. Every word of that news column was soothing my heart as I was correlating with the age.

I showed it to Soni, "look at this column."

She replied, "You should learn from her."

I said, "I am feeling bad that I didn't care for my baby till now."

She said, "It's ok."

Now, I have started admiring this gift. Though my house and health situations are not very good but still I promised myself to give my baby a good life. From that day, I started caring for myself so that my baby remained safe and ignored the age thing.

The news of baby comes with a lot of changes in our life. Poverty started disappearing. Karan's income got increased. We got TV, cooler, inverter and many more basic essentials in our home.I didn't consider the baby a lucky charm because of this but because I had got my life back again and baby gave me a purpose in life. No matter how many times one experience pregnancy but every new baby comes with new vibes, having their own ways to fascinate their mom. The little kicks in stomach still feels fascinating. Back in those days, we didn't used to go to clinics for check up but my mind always kept enquiring about the health of the baby, "if baby is weak due to my age or if baby is getting enough food or not or, if baby's body is paining when my body used to pain or, if baby is feeling cold as I am feeling cold". All the feelings used to make me really tensed.

One day, while I was sitting near the door, one of the oldest and most experienced woman of our society was roaming outside and she came to me to ask about the baby.

I told her, "I hope baby is ok".

She then told me, "Baby is coming late, maybe to bring happiness for you". Her words relaxed me.

The three trimesters went by in the same manner and the day had come when I gave birth to a baby girl. I used to admire goddess Gayatri a lot so, I gave her name 'Gayatri'.

The doctor informed, "The baby is healthy but too small, just 2 kgs."

I asked in tension, "Will the weight have any side effects if she is very weak?"

Doctor consoled me not to worry and also told to take proper rest and take care of the little one.

I am glad to have conceived my daughter in my late forties. Atleast, due to improved financial conditions, I was able to give her a good life, proper education and flowered her well.

*****

"Ask a child how it feels to live without a person to love, care and sacrifice and then tell me again, no one loves you?"

~Priyanshi Mussadi

Inception Of Angel

~Mala Nirola

So we sat in front of the doctor and kept our fingers crossed. My heart pounded and looking meekly at Sameer, I held his hands tightly. He responded by patting the back of my palms with adoration and pressed them gently between his palms. Yes, I had missed my periods and we decided to get an Elisa test done which instantly gave us the report. It was positive. Our happiness knew no bounds but the doctor had to examine first.

After the doctor's confirmation, we got certain tests done. I was advised few do's and don'ts, medicines prescribed and the EDD (expected date of delivery) was given. I was asked to get few blood tests, HIV, Rh factor, pressure , sugar etc done. I was advised to take proper diets and do exercises regularly. That was how my daughter made us feel her presence in this world.

Days went by, when one morning as I was getting ready to go to school, the spices from the kitchen didn't smell as aromatic as I usually found them to be, instead, I found it nauseating. The next moment, I felt giddy, so I held Sameer's shoulder from back for support and what happened next was all that Sameer had narrated to me later. He said that I had almost lost my consciousness. He lifted me by his arms and laid me on the bed. Our landlady who was a staff nurse in the government hospital immediately came for my rescue. She guided us well. Soon the news of my pregnancy spread like wildfire from my parents to my in-laws to their relatives, my colleagues and friends and also to the landlady's relatives.

The advises, needless to say, started flooding in, uninvited and free. Many asked what I wanted to eat or if I had any special craving for, whether I had morning or evening sickness and many such volleys of questions. But frankly speaking, I neither had any special craving then nor did I experience any sickness. I would eat anything to everything. I ate in the morning, at noon in the evening and again a bowlful of food at night. Sweets were always a way to reward myself. This does not include the list of fruits, nuts, snacks, chips and many other things that I binged on all times.

I was told that pregnancy was not easy as it came with mood swings, morning and evening sickness, pressure shooting up, pain, swelling, nausea and many such things but except for mild giddiness almost every day, I faced no major problem. Not even once, at least in the first four to five months. I ate, slept, walked, shopped, worked everything with ease.

I attended my work regularly as usual and time went by. I started going for walks and did few simple exercises too. Soon, we visited the doctor as it was the end of the third month and I had entered into the second trimester.

At the beginning of the second trimester, I had no problem at all. It was same as the first three months. It was only towards the end of the fifteenth week, when I realised, I did not like the smell coming out from the kitchen. The smell of spices, oils, rice ,*chapati* or anything irked me. So, Sameer had taken charge of the kitchen fully. Sometimes even the smell of boiling milk made me feel puckish.

By the end of the eighteenth week, I had to get the first USG done. The thought and the feeling was eternal as I was going to have the first glance of my baby. The USG report was shown to my doctor who looked satisfied and said "Baby is developing well, all is good!".As usual, he scribbled on his note pad some medicines; some were new and some had to be repeated and a series of tests to be done again.

By the end of the second trimester, I started feeling uneasy while sleeping sideways. I had to keep tossing, so I had started keeping oblong cotton stuffed huge pillow for support in between my legs. I slept with it throughout in the remaining period of my pregnancy. My belly had started protruding and I could see and feel the little life trying to make itself comfortable in its compact world. That was the time when I felt its first "kick".

The crucial third trimester had begun and the doctor once again advised me to do all sort of activities that I did in regular basis but refrain from travelling long distances. I had no problem to that. Within a month, the belly had become very large. I used to feel starved at all times. I remember, once I got up at 2 am feeling thirsty and ended up eating an apple and two bananas. I could no longer hide my belly under my *shawl* or *dupatta.* It was open for display. My weight had substantially increased. Fine stretch marks began to appear in and around the belly and the thighs. The breasts became large and the hands and feet began to swell. I was advised to lessen the salt intake. The blood sugar, pressure and other tests became very frequent as the D-day was approaching. We did quick shopping of basic stuff like baby blankets, baskets, cradle and other things. My mother came and took charge of the house now. I had not stopped from going to work although simple activities like bending in front, tossing and turning, clipping toe-nails , bathing, tying strings of the petticoat, picking objects from the floor became a difficult job. I had to widen my feet to walk with ease as it gave the proper grip to the floor. Sameer said I walked like a duck. I had already stopped wearing heels as comfortable flat sandals had replaced them.

I continued to go to work till my last day as I had no problem in doing other day to day activities. I even attended a wedding ceremony on my delivery date.

Five days went past my **EDD** and still I had no indication like pain or whatsoever. It was one of my colleagues who forcibly admitted me to the hospital and thus ten days after the date of delivery I was induced pain which proved fruitless. Finally the next day, through C-section, my little angel came to this world and I became mother of a cuddly, cute, beautiful, healthy princess weighing 3.9kg

*****

> *"It's like happiness is knocking at the door when a baby kicks in uterus"*
>
> **~Sadaf Rehan**

Gift Of Grace

~*Joyeeta Roy*

A married woman feels complete when she embraces motherhood. God has bestowed women with immense power and strength to carry within her another life. As the embryo passes through various stages, so does the expecting mother. She not only goes through physical and hormonal changes but psychological changes too. She prepares herself mentally to welcome a new member who would make its advent into this harsh yet beautiful world.

Nine months of physical strain, mental stress and display of fortitude is what goes into the making of a mother. My life has gone through a lot of turmoil and I believed that a child could be the only source of appeasement for me. To add to my woes, I discovered that I was unable to conceive.

After undergoing treatment for a few months, to my surprise I conceived which was difficult to believe. I felt ecstatic. It was nothing but the grace of God.

Thus, began my journey of carrying that tiny seed of life through the three trimesters which was not cakewalk at all. In fact, the first trimester was a tight rope walk. Any mother at this stage needs to be the most careful. A little carelessness could spoil the whole story. I remember the doctors warning me against any kind of movement during the 1st trimester. That could enhance the risk of the foetus being dislodged from the womb and losing it forever.

Morning sickness is one of the earliest symptoms of pregnancy and I was not spared too. It was awful waking up with a nauseating feeling. But the moment I remembered that tiny life is growing inside me, all uneasiness disappeared.   Losing one's appetite was another problem to be dealt with seriously because it was important for a would - be mother to eat well but right after conceiving, I was hit hard by it. The very mention of food made me sick. The smell of spices and curries was enough to trigger nausea. I tried all kinds of food, spoiling myself with choices but all I did was just nibble and leave unfinished.

The first month of the first trimester was indeed very troublesome but after that, things were much better. Gradually, in the next two months, all the initial symptoms disappeared. Thoughts about the baby kept me engrossed most of the time. As I entered the second trimester, I could feel the changes that my body was undergoing. It was making space for my bundle of joy which made its presence felt every moment inconspicuously. Sometimes I felt overpowered by my growing emotions, apprehensions , speculations, etc. Would I give birth to a healthy child? Would I be able to manage my child? Many such questions filled me with anxiety. But I tried to keep my mind diverted by reading books, my unfailing companion and also listening to some good music. I hoped that it would reach my baby too.

During second semester, my baby bump became noticeable and many of my friends and acquaintances who did not know about my pregnancy got the shock of their life. It was beyond their imagination that I would ever experience motherhood, considering the negative test results earlier with no ray of hope. And now this was like sunshine for me and my loved ones too basked in it.

Six months seemed to pass in a jiffy. I entered the third trimester. Now I was in my seventh month. This last semester was very crucial. I had to be very careful. Carrying a growing baby in the womb for six long months and more was nothing less than climbing a mountain but despite all discomfort; the movement of the little one inside made me forget everything. His kicks and stunts were enough to lighten my mood and fill me with exuberance. A baby shower was thrown by my mother-in-law and it was quite fun participating in the rituals which were associated with the well being of my unborn baby.

Visiting the doctor every month for a rigorous check-up was a ritual too which had to be followed strictly and an USG (ultra-sonography) was also a must in order to know how the baby was doing, like if it's growth was normal, if there was any kind of abnormality and many such critical and scary things which made my heart skip a beat every time I went for it. Thankfully, things were normal. During this last semester, in the eighth month again I had to go for an USG, which was probably the last one. When I saw the image of the baby, I was overwhelmed with joy. It was a fully grown baby now, almost ready to push itself out, just a matter of another month.

I now entered the last month of the last trimester. Nine long months of wait would soon be over. I still vividly remember the tentative date of delivery given by the doctor. It was 10th Feb 2000. As I neared this date, I was gripped by nervousness. I did not want to go for caesarean at all and my doctor too convinced me that he won't go for it unless the situation called for.

It was 8th Feb and I started experiencing pain in my abdomen since morning. I was sure my labor pain had started and immediately I called up my doctor. He advised me to get admitted as soon as possible and we wasted no time. After I got myself admitted, my baby and I were being closely monitored. Everything was normal but there was no sign of the baby trying to push itself out. The doctors said that it was 'false labor pain' and I was sent back home the next day, highly disappointed.

Finally, on 19th February, I went into labor and the intense, painful and frequent contractions lasted one whole night. I writhed and wriggled in pain but it was worth it. On 20th February, early in the morning, my little prince made a royal entry into our lives. It was a normal delivery and the pain that I went through was indescribable but just a look at the baby, who was my flesh and blood, was enough to erase all pain.

At every step, life teaches us a lesson. I learnt the best lesson of my life through the birth of my child. Our life is beset with pain and hardships which are not everlasting. Good and happy times always follow which help us forget those turbulent times. This is the essence of life.

*****

> *"The mother is the best invention of God, which means mind-blowing, outstanding, true, honest, energetic and reliable star performer in life's all tasks"*
>
> ~Manisha Goyal

Persistence Of Hope

~Sunita Chaudhary

One year had not passed away of my marriage and I came to know that I was going to be a "Mother." It was the month of October "2002". I still remember the time, when, at my home our family doctor had come and done the pregnancy test and the report was positive. Everyone in my family was happy, yet we decided to visit the doctor for regular checkups on next day, for the self satisfaction. And the next day all the test took place and the report was definitely positive again. That was a moment of happiness. Because, I was going to be a mother for the first time. I was having no experience yet as I was only 21 years old. My husband, mother -in-law, father – in – law and everyone in our family had supported me.

Now medicines and precautions were given by the doctor to me and they were my responsibilities. I was asked to come for routine check-ups. One month passed away very quietly. Now, it was the month of November and vomit, nausea started. My husband instantly called the doctor, and then doctor prescribed me. I went for regular checkups as per doctor's prescription. In the third month, doctor had given me medication. Now blood test, blood pressure, body weight were checked timely. A feeling of satiation took place that I was going to be a mother. I was asked to drink as much water as I can and to sleep in a proper way for the better development of baby.

It was my mother in law who helped me in all the works of home especially in bathing during gestation period. My husband and father-in-law were taking care of my diet by giving me essential meals like- fresh fruits and all the food as suggested by the doctor to me. In the fourth and fifth month, apart from nutritious food I was asked to include fruits, nuts, cashew, almonds, raisins and homemade juices of orange and all. During this period whenever I watched television, I used to listen Dr. A.P.J Abdul Kalam's speech , Atal Bihari Vajpayee and *"Aap Ki Aadalat"* show of Mr. Rajat Sharma. Also Movies of Bollywood legends like Amitabh Bachchan and Rajnikant, in order to have a positive impact of these famous personalities on my baby.

In the sixth month, I began to feel the movement made by the baby. Yet during this period, itching occurred in my stomach and to remain calm and careful during the situation, I had to do it with a cloth and not by hands. I was asked to eat cashews after soaking them in water. Pomegranate is that fruit which I had always taken. I was asked not to eat spinach, brinjal in order to prevent the baby from infection. In the seventh and eighth month, baby started moving completely in the stomach. I started talking with the baby. Several thoughts surrounded my mind like "When the baby will say me mother...?" I decided that I would serve my baby the best . I would explain everything to the baby as a friend. No matter what the baby would be – a girl or a boy. I would treat both the same.

As it was the summer season, so sweating was a part. I drank much water and ate juicy fruits – watermelon and all for better development of my baby. I was asked not to eat *jalebis* , though I liked it. The doctor had given me the date of 2nd June but there were no signs for the birth of baby, so, I didn't go to the doctor. On June 4, 2003 at 9am, my stomach started paining. I hadn't informed it to anyone in the family. I hadn't told about it to anyone in my family and completed my daily work as usual. But in the afternoon the pain was at the highest. I couldn't even bear it. I realized that the baby was about to be born. I informed it to my husband and mother-in-law. They took me to the government hospital. We reached there around 6pm. The doctor examined me and said "No". To be very honest I was worried about my baby.

"Why the doctor said no...?"

This question prevailed in my mind again and again. Yet I didn't lose hope. Now, I was taken to private doctor, Mr. Manoj Agarwal where his wife,Dr.Himani Agarwal examined me and said "Yes, the baby is going to born." I was overwhelmed from inside. And as soon as possible, I was admitted to the hospital's "operation room" I think it was around 8 pm. And suddenly, doctors put there all scary tools in front of me. I was surrounded by lady doctor and nurses. Pain was much high, yet, I forgot everything. My eyes were still struck on the wall clock. At around 9pm,doctor said "thrust on". I, with my whole effort, put the pressure and I felt like something round was coming out. Again the doctor said thrust on. I made the effort. After sometime my stomach was empty. I felt relaxed.

At last that moment came for which I was waiting since last 9 months, the baby started crying. Then, I was taken to another room where the nurse cleaned my private parts and after that I was given a bed where I rested. The nurse came around 9:45 pm, holding my baby in her hands and she informed me that "A girl is born". I was very happy to hear that. She further informed me "Today 11 babies born in the hospital in total. The rest 10 are boys and the 11th one is this girl. When we saw your round stomach we thought that a boy was going to born again but it came to be a girl."

Not only my family members and relatives were happy but the whole staff of that hospital was happy at the birth of my baby girl. Everyone congratulated my husband and he distributed the sweets in the hospital. Dr.Himani Agarwal, with the nurse came to me and the nurse gave a cloth and a nipple for the baby. Further, Dr.Himani Agarwal came and praised me by saying "Every mother has to bear this pain but you are courageous, you didn't tremble." I was very happy to hear this because I can bear any pain for my baby.

I am feeling blessed that I am able to share this life experience journey of being a mother first time.

*****

"If you think love is ending from your life, then hail to your mother and she can pour your whole life with love and happiness"

~Abhishek Rai

Core Of Existence

~Lamiya Siraj

Finally, the day came in my life with the help of which, in future, I would be known as complete. Much awaited day after being married for seven long years. Had been waiting for five years to see '+ve' sign on my pregnancy test kit. Right after two years of marriage I was getting bombarded with the question "When are you giving the good news?" Initially we were able to take this question and use to revert it with a smile but soon it took a toll on us and got converted into frustration. Every day became a torture for us until August 2008.

I had missed my menstrual cycle and had decided to undergo the test once again (though it was very painful for me, as by now, I had forgotten the count for how many times I have taken this test and disappointed myself with negative results.) Still praying hard and attracting all positive energies from universe keeping myself calm, I took the test. I couldn't believe myself after I saw my result. My 1st reaction after the test showed I am pregnant was "WOW!" Am I pregnant? Is it true? After a couple of tests (to confirm the news), I was ecstatic. Happiness had no bounds. Me and my husband were on the top of the world.

Before I understood, morning sickness started. It started with week 8 and lasted till week 15. It did stay for the whole day, but mornings were bad, very bad! I was left with no other choice but to keep puke bags, packed tissues and orange candy all the time with me. I was recommended complete bed rest for my 1st trimester as I was bleeding continuously. I felt ravenous, then nauseous. This got over only in the 2nd trimester. During my scan, seeing this 8-week-old foetus on screen, it's tiny heart beating, was one of the most unforgettable moment of my life. I realised it's a life, living inside my body. This was one-day-at-a-time type of adventure.

For me, my second trimester of pregnancy is one of the best phases of my pregnancy. I no more felt nauseated and fatigue. I had my husband by my side always, loving and comforting me.I had started feeling comfortable and my appetite was back. I was getting compliments about my skin that it's glowing. My baby bump was now visible. I had started feeling a new set of experiences. I could feel changes in my skin and had started developing stretch marks.

I still remember the gush of emotions on my husband's face when we had gone for the ultrasound scan during my 22nd week and had visualized the baby. With the help of doctor, we were able to see the overall development of our baby and were relieved about its wellbeing. For me, it was important that as a father, he creates a sense of bonding during second trimester.

Now started the tough times and difficult days of my life. Sleeping became difficult for me. No position while sleeping was giving me comfort. I used to wake my husband up every couple of hours to help me turn over and to help me off the bed every time I wanted to go to washroom. I had developed a phobia and was getting hell scared each time when I didn't feel the move of my baby for more than 15 mins. I had formed a habit of talking with my baby. Telling stories and sharing the real incidents of life. Also, I was making my baby aware of immediate family members. I felt an intense protectiveness towards my baby. I was very scared of actual birth part since starting. But more than that I feared losing the baby for any reason before birth. With my anxiety and sleep deprivation, I had formed a habit to soothing myself and started a brisk walk every night with my husband. He not only understood me well but also supported me with all my mood swings and health problems. He was very calm and composed. We were counting days now for our baby to arrive in this world. The best part for both of us was 'kicking'. I had felt 1ˢᵗ kick of my baby in afternoon when he was at office. Since then I was waiting for him to come and feel it. But our baby was naughty before birth and knew how to tease parents. We waited whole evening, till late night but nothing happened. Finally, my husband was able to feel baby's first kick in the early morning next day. Baby used to kick me in the ribs or in the crotch. It's an intriguing experience.

The best part for this trimester was 'shopping'. It was our first child, so we didn't want to know the gender though we were curious. We wanted to keep it secret till the last on GOD's wish. But shopping was important and necessary items were essential, so it became more exciting for us what to buy and how to buy. We tried getting unisex items as much as possible.

Starting of week 36, we had our final visit to the doctor. Due to few complications the day was finalized for our little one to arrive in this world, into our lives and make us complete, making me 'whole'. My hospital bag was ready and lying below the bed for more than a week before my last visit to doctor for any emergency. I still remember the labor room. The scariest table which takes legs in air, but still the most needed one. Finally, the day arrived. It was that morning 8:27 am, 15ᵗʰ April 2009, Wednesday when I first heard the cry of my little angel. It was a baby girl declared by my doctor. There were no limits of my happiness as I always have prayed and wanted a daughter. A companion for my life. Doctor took her and immediately kept her on my chest. The heart beats that I was hearing till date through ultrasound machine was in real now. I was able to hear it, feel it. Tears of joy were flowing continuously from my eyes. I had forgotten all my pain. Happiness had taken over it. Suddenly I felt all my pain has vanished.

I had my life in my hand. Our bundle of joy. Feeling of tiny finger holding my finger was the most divine and unforgettable moment of my life.

I would like to end my experience of 3 trimesters of my life here by stating,
"Giving birth is a new birth for the mothers even!"

*****

"Confront well before everyone but stop for a while when it's about your mom"

~Shweta Padole

Medallion Of Womb

~Nahid Khanam

I was hitched at a tender age when I was still learning from books. I finished my graduation and after three years of togetherness, we planned our first child. But it was not as easy as I was imagining. My husband used to stay in another city. We spent eleven months with no positive results. I was 20years old. I gave up hope and started thinking that maybe I have some problem. I was anaemic. So, I decided to carry on my education. I got admission in MA. But in just three months of my Masters degree I conceived. I skipped my period. And the special card confirmed my pregnancy. I gave this news to my husband and he was very happy. But then I had to decide whether to continue my study or to drop out. My husband supported and encouraged me a lot in my journey. I continued to study but took leave from classes. And thus, my journey to a new world started.

I was vomiting a lot and it resulted in low consumption of food. Headache, mood swings and back pain were my inseparable companions. I lost nearly 5 to 6kgs. It was terrifying. But feeling butterflies in your belly is such blissful that you forget about all and just smile. Everyone in the family was more than happy. Frequent check-ups and my gynaecologist helped me a lot.

The first sonography confirmed that I was having single foetus in my womb. I was adviced bed rest by the doctor. Yoga, morning walk and intake of more water were unavoidable. I maintained balance between my pregnancy and study. Because my exam schedule and ultrasound confirmed that I can appear for my second semester during the last month of my pregnancy.

Being an anaemic, my blood pressure remained low that caused drowsiness all the time. But nights were sleepless. Funny part was that, after 28 weeks I stopped vomiting but I was peeing in and after every 15 minutes. I was suffering from constipation, severe back pain. My mother was a constant support to me.

Finally, I completed 30weeks. Now my baby had started kicking and turning. I could see movement over my skin. And that feeling can't be expressed in words. Sometimes my eyes were full of tears. I was carrying a life within myself. I am a dreamer. I was imagining how I would take care of my baby. I used to talk to my abdomen. My blood group is negative. This also became a reason of my anxiety. Sometimes I was very panicked. Without any reason I felt like crying. I talked to the doctor and she said all this was because of pregnancy.

I completed 32weeks. My semester started. I was not even able to sit. Everyone in the family advised me to skip the examination as I had to sit and write for four hours continuously. On the other hand my mother and husband encouraged me that I can do it. Nevertheless I completed my examination. But my complexity increased. When we reached home from exam centre I was having unbearable pain. We contacted to doctor. She recommended sonography. But I was not being able to tolerate the pain. I cried whole night.

The next morning I was admitted to the hospital. Nurse said that pain was not enough for vaginal birth. My amniotic sac had low water level and baby was distress. I was crying and wondering if my baby was going to be fine. I was cursing myself. They tried to induce labor tolerance. My baby's head was big and I dilated only 2cm. Water bag broke and bleeding started. I fainted. Doctor told my family to take decision immediately; if they would go with caesarean section because I needed urgent operation.

I broke down when my sister hugged me saying, "Everything is gonna fine. Have faith on Allah." I felt like I'm going to die. I panicked. I told the doctor "I hadn't asked for apologies what if I die." Doctor tried to assure me saying, "nothing wrong will happen dear." She injected me with anaesthesia. I heard voice of my baby crying. I could see everyone around me when I was shifted to my bed from OT. And then I got unconscious. After hours, when I got back my senses I asked Ammi about my baby. Ammi said it's a girl. "My darling smile, Allah blessed us with an angel. Now you are also a mother," she said.

My complications didn't end here. I hadn't eaten for three days and I was given double doses of anaesthesia that induced gastritis and longer drowsiness. My baby also suffered from this. Doctor advised me not to feed the baby for 6 to 7hours. I was shattered, feeling like a cursed mother who was not being able to feed her child but pouring milk and throwing in to the wastage. Medication helped me in healing faster.

On 5th day, I was discharged and we returned back to home. After all these struggles, hurdles broke down when I saw the heavenly reward I felt the celestial bliss. I was overwhelmed with happiness. Holding the baby and seeing her feeding, the tiny soft movement of her lips and fingers, I forgot all the hustle and smiled. My scars smiled. My angel engraved a permanent smile on me.

*****

> *"The world's most pleasant pain is felt by the womb which carries the life"*
>
> *~Talima Das*

Joy Of Glutton

~*Aarthy R.*

The day I missed my girly days I was excited and surprised at the same time. I was looking forward to the moment of being a "Mom" for almost a year. I wanted to take this slow and confirm things. I waited for another month and a half and there came "The Big News". I am going to be a mom. I never knew two red lines could bring such a big joy to my family. Hence, started my first trimester.

I was abroad in a different country and working, my family was worried about me being alone, since it's my first baby. I didn't know what to do and what not to do. I took baby steps to understand what this whole pregnancy thing is all about. It's not just about mom and baby, it's about the bonding of the family. I knew, I am pregnant but I didn't feel a thing. I was very curious about how my little one is doing. There came a doctor consultation on my 10th-week that's nearing the end of my first trimester. The doctor examined me and said that I am in good health and poor in Vitamin D which is usually low in Asian moms and I am ok to go through the fun ride. She gave me a small piece of scan sheet showing my little one.

Nothing could explain that moment and tears rolled down and I still don't have words to explain how I felt. I took care of myself well by taking more hygienic food and almost vegetables all the time. It gives the baby good nourishment. I started reading good books to keep my thoughts positive and started meditating too. I wanted to give all good things to my little one as far as I can. I stopped eating too hot food as I heard that it might not be good for babies. Days of getting used to medium-hot food. I also started communicating with my baby from the 10th-week though I didn't care about whether it reached my little one or not. I wanted to explain things that happen around me and have a little child and mom time daily.

In the second Trimester, I decided to move back home so that I could feel the warmth of home and native. After 20 weeks, as that's the best time Airline allows you along with your official work from home and maternal holiday options. Yes, you heard it right, it's not called leave its holiday I would be enjoying my maternity. Even during the second check-up, doctor was a bit suspicious as I never gained weight instead, I had lost some. She asked me to get one checkup on the 18th-week. I was worried as I couldn't felt any of the kicks like other moms and felt a bit depressed. I waited for the 18th-week to come so that I could see my little one on big screen. My little one was so shy and active. My little one turned around a lot and it became so hard for the examiner to take proper snapshots. Finally, after 18 minutes of rolling down struggle we got a wonderful video and pic of my little one growing up healthy. The doctor was also surprised that the baby was in good health despite my loss of weight. I was so happy that day I called each and everyone in my family to show how active and healthy my little one was. I was overwhelmed in the joy of motherhood and it's exactly 21st-week when I felt my little one's first kick according to the records. I started listening to good music and I could feel the kicks in response. We had our own music time and communication time, longer now than before. I was worried about 18 hours over a flight but then Airlines gave such good care and helped me land safely at home. Roads to the village might be longer but then again I entered my home at 2 AM. Because of time zone difference, my mom had prepared me food at such midnight hours so that I may feel nourished with my little one. I carried all the reports as I had to switch doctor because of relocation. I visited the new one and she also said that I and my little one were perfectly fine.

Last trimester started and so did the biweekly checkups. Though I was enjoying my moments, thrill and fear combined in my heart started while the days were approaching. I was afraid of the pain I would go through and the pain my little one would go through to come out. I spoke a lot about meeting each other soon and in response got kicks as usual. I was working 6 hours a day by then. My mom would take me on walks and let me do small household chores as it would help my pregnancy. I had my 27th-week check-up and things were still fine. I continued my diets with more liquid food supplements made of lentils and vegetables and had decent walks along the street. I collaborated with everyone and learned multiple things about being "Mom".

On my 32nd week, I had another pic of my little one added to the album. I was continuing my work from home for 4 hours a day. Things were on smooth sail till 34th-week. All of a sudden my water broke and I didn't know what has happened and I gave a loud cry and my mom and relatives rushed me to hospital. I was crying and was afraid that something would happen to my little one and all I could think was about my little one and I never had myself in mind. Later I realized that's the selflessness any mother would inculcate unknowingly. They gave me injections to reduce pain but of no help and I was rushed to operation theatre as per procedures. I was given an injection and they were taking my little one out and I was half-conscious when I heard my little one cry. Wow... I now knew that my little one has arrived in this world and I am the person whom my little one would look out for. I slowly went into a deep sleep. By the time when I woke up, they had already transferred me to the general ward and my little one was awake too. I felt like my little one was waiting for me to wake up. They made me turn around slowly since I was being operated and placed my little one covered in blue on me. The first touch of me, my little one kicked again. I felt the bond within and my little should have felt the same too. That's how my three trimesters for life got concluded.

*****

> *"Mothers are like heavenly angels and that heaven without those angels seems unfair and likewise a home without mothers will make one's life incomplete, unhappy"*
>
> *~Muhamad Asarudeen .S*

Drizzle Of Mercy

~Huda Farooq

In the patient wait of 7 years to watch the second pink line appear on the pregnancy test kit, there were moments which shattered me, there were words that scared me, there were hopes that abandoned me, yet, if I was able to remain strong and take all of them with a smile, it was because of my unwavering faith in the fate written by the Almighty. I was hurt but wasn't broken, I was worried but wasn't disheartened. I was scared but wasn't devastated. And then one fine morning, in the September of 2016, my faith triumphed as the lifeless pregnancy kit finally announced the existence of a life within me.

From there began a journey of unexplainable bliss, the 3 trimesters for life.

I remember how nervous I was until the doctor read from my Beta HCG report and confirmed that I was 4 weeks pregnant. '4 weeks! Is that all?' I had asked her impatiently, wishing I had discovered my pregnancy a little later, as I would have to wait for another 35 weeks or so to hold my little bundle of joy in my arms. I sounded stupid to my own ears when the doctor chuckled and I realized what I had said. On the way back home, I realized I was not the only stupid person here, when my husband exclaimed "Why does the baby take so long to come into this world? Can't it come sooner?" I giggled at his impatient remark and said "You have waited for 7 years. How hard it is for you to wait for another 8 months?" He replied "That wait was different from this." I nodded my head with a huge grin and affirmed that my feelings were not different.

My first trimester was not less than a cakewalk. My biggest relief was that I did not suffer from morning sickness and that's the very reason why all other unusual changes in me seemed trivial to me. I enormously enjoyed being pampered by people around me. While my mother and my sister were at my beck and call, my husband had become extra cautious and over-protective for me - although I groaned about it at times, yet I enjoyed his attention and loved this side of him. My best friend at my workplace would every day, delight me with a delicious breakfast (rather call it a meal). 'Perks of being pregnant' you see!

If pregnancy brings along a bunch of happiness, it also comes with a bundle of worries. It would not be wrong to term pregnancy as the most uncertain period of waiting in life. You can never predict when and what will go wrong, and that fear keeps looming over your head throughout the journey. The detection of the fetal heartbeat was one such big fear I had. Although my faith in the fate was strong enough to assure me, the fear that came with it was unignorable. I literally felt my heart in my mouth, until I was able to hear my child's heartbeat in the 12th week's scan. The moment the resonant sound echoed in the silent dark room and hit my ears, I felt ecstatic and my heartbeats seemed to rhyme and synchronize with my child's heartbeat, I could hear them beating at a rate faster than usual.

As I stepped into the second trimester, I had to discard some of my favorite clothes that I had been wearing for ages. I am sure mom must have been elated that I finally put them away. I ditched the traditional drawstring *salwars* and opted for the comfortable elastic band pajamas. I got too comfortable with the latter that till date I have not been able to go back to wearing the former.

My bestie, one day, exclaimed, "Weeks seem to fly by!"

"Nope," I quipped immediately disagreeing with her. "Days pass by faster but weeks are moving at a snail's space," I added.

"How is that even possible? You are contradicting your own words," she said.

"Believe me! I was 14 weeks far last weekend and I am still 14 weeks and 5 days far today," I groaned. She grinned finding my impatience 'cute'.

Weeks somehow passed and my excitement started growing as I stepped into the 8th month of my pregnancy. A shocking discovery awaited us when we visited the doctor. The growth of my baby was getting slower and my cervix had begun funneling, which meant that I could go into a pre-mature labor. I was advised complete bed rest. Everyone at home was worried for me and a few people even tried to implant the fear that I may not be able to deliver a healthy baby. Amidst all the worries and fears, I felt my faith in the fate strengthening and I knew that if I have come so far, I will be able to hold a healthy baby in my arms soon.

2 weeks ahead of my expected due date, the doctor discovered that the amniotic fluid levels were decreasing, and the growth of the baby seemed to have stilled. I was admitted that very night and the doctors tried to induce labor. After the 3rd induction and 36 hours of waiting in the labor room, when there was no desired progress in my condition, the doctors decided to do a C-section. Placing my faith in what was willed for me, I

signed the consent form and was taken into the OT in a few hours. The feeling of being pushed into the OT on a stretcher was scary and I had chills running down my spine. I was then lying on the operating table, conscious but voluntarily blocking my senses to what was going on around me until my senses were awakened with the first cry of my baby. If I had felt that the sound of my baby's first heartbeat was most enthralling, the first cry was far more fascinating. The nurse brought my baby close to my face and mentioned it's a girl. I just leaned forward and kissed her on the cheek and my lips curved to form the biggest smile of my life.

'Our daughter!', I and my husband hummed elatedly. Yes, we finally had someone whom we could call 'ours'. She was undoubtedly an answer to our prayers, the mercy of the Almighty, the precious gift from God. So, we named her 'Inaayah' which means 'a blessing of God'.

"Jaane kiski dua thi jo qubool hui
Ke Rab ki mujhpe ye INAAYATH hui"

*****

"From the sleepless nights to constant worries, a mother is always ready to try best for her children"

~Dimple Rohra

Quest Of Maternity

~Arshiya Patel

A magical time in life after a certain phase of "Marriage", Everyone desires to live this moment. The moment came in my life after a year and was so quick to understand.

Quest to embark the scoop

One evening, we had been to the park, roaming hand in hand talking about random stuffs and enjoying the joyous breeze and out of nowhere, a ball came flying and hit my stomach so hard for a moment I felt blank. Group of boys playing football came running and apologized for their actions.

After two to three days, I got severe stomach pain. We rushed to the doctor, she asked me about what happened. Then to my surprise, she said I'm expecting .I was baffled between about how to say this glad little tiding to my better half. And in a matter of time, we both were staring at each other's eyes filled with utter emotions. All I 'could feel was gratitude, compassion and pride.

The journey so far was not manageable, nor bearable, to say it was very tough. But, with constant support and wishes from my husband and family, I was able to complete this journey.

The first phase:

Vomiting, change of mood, nausea, irritation became constant as the weeks of pregnancy progressed.
Every time when I vomited, my husband would come running with a piece of lemon in his hand. Weird cravings for *Bhatkaly*

food, biryani was what I get in middle of nowhere. My pregnancy was typical, with full of workload and uneventful for 9 months.

Demeanor with Emotions

In my second month of pregnancy, I started feeling nausea, and dizziness. My husband took care of me like a small child ,no matter how much I irritated him he just used to smile .Every time he used to leave for work, he used to say,"Had your breakfast?, Good, see ya Luv," and he used to flew out the door.

Regularly visiting hospital became my routine for the next 4 months. By Almighty's grace, I got the opportunity to visit Mecca. But, the doctor had strictly told me not to travel, but I wanted to perform umrah.

I performed pilgrimage in the fourth month of my pregnancy. There were a lot of hurdles, people telling, "You won't be able to perform umrah, look at you, you have become so weak and all that stuffs." Heedlessness to what they were saying, I took my baby as my strength and went to perform Umrah. By the grace of Almighty, I performed it with ease.

In few days,I had my first ultrasound. We all knew that in foreign countries doctors used to reveal the gender. Luckily, I was abroad with my hubby at that time.

The second phase:

My first scan was at my 5th month and there they were going to reveal the gender of the baby. We were so much curious to know the gender. So, during my regular check-up in the fifth month, Doctor led me to a dark room, asked me to lay on the bed as she was investigating. I saw my husband peeping through the curtain, then the doctor asked him to come inside and he was looking at the monitor. He was amazed to see the baby's traces in the monitor. He made eye contact with me and said to ask the gender, there was an intense silence, but, after a few minutes she said, "It's a **BOY**." Yes, I heard, it is a boy. He was very happy. He was hoping for a "Boy".

Till the second phase of my pregnancy, I was in abroad with my husband. I missed my family badly. I badly wanted to sleep in my mother's lap. I was suffering a lot, yes my husband was there, supported me in this phase, still, I was feeling homesick, regularly I used to video call my family, but that wasn't satisfying me. But, Almighty gave me the strength to deal with all this pain. And the time came when I had to leave for India. It was very hard, really hard to leave him and go back as my visa was expiring.

The third phase:

I had severe headaches, sore feet and nausea up to 7 months. I was back in India after 6 months. Oh! I missed my college, as I was pursuing my bachelor of education, so I had to go to college. My college was located on the cliff where there were no auto or canteen facilities. But my batchmates were kind enough to help me in fulfilling my food carvings. It was my last semester of B.ed. It was full of assignments and teachings methods.

World at My arms

These 3 phases of life was not easy, rather say, it was topsy turvy. Every phase taught me how to overcome emotions and pain taught me to accept every situation as a part of life. Blessing in disguise suits exactly right for this phase of life.

No matter what you withhold during this phase, in the end, you hold little tiny lad, who will mean the world to you.
At that very moment, you forget everything you bore just to hold this tiny existence of you .At that moment, I learned how to smile when you are in pain.

It's giving new life and getting a new life.

*****

"All of the lies and unspoken words that your heart is holding, can be read out like an open book by a mother's mind"

~Ayushi Sharma

Revival Of Spirit

~Tasneem Fatima

My journey to motherhood started after 4 years of my marriage. It was the most memorable and beautiful day of my life when I got to know that 'I'm pregnant'. Now that I'm the mother of a 2 year old toddler, when I look back to those days when I was expecting it feels like I'm the bravest woman in the world to go through all of it.

The first trimester was full of excitement and cravings. Nevertheless to mention, it was tiring and exhausting too. Because of continuous restless nights and the feeling of puking all the time(which turns into truth most of the time).But all this struggle and health issues got overpowered with the feeling of holding your baby in your arms in a few months, and dreaming about having a third cute and tiny member in the family.

In my second scan, I could hear the heartbeat of my baby. I cried out of joy. It was overwhelming to feel two hearts beating inside me. Every scan I went through made me thrilled and emotional to see that tiny creature growing eventually.

The first trimester passed very fast. When the 5th month started, I could literally feel something moving inside. It had become my favourite hobby to put my hand on my belly and wait for the baby to move or give a kick. But at the same time, I couldn't sleep properly at any time of the day or night. Sleepless nights made me restless. I craved sweets so much that my sugar level increased instantly. Doctor immediately asked me to stop eating anything sugary and to avoid sweets. I loved going for walks and taking fresh breaths. My favourite spot at that time was the colony park. And my favourite liquid which I had a lot was "*nariyal paani.*"

Then came the last trimester with a lot of struggle, stress and health issues. Although, I was excited and waiting for this time of my pregnancy, I did not expect all these problems to arise. I suffered from iron deficiency. I had to take the Iron via IV. My thyroid level abruptly changed and I had to go through tests and change the medicines.

This was the time I could see the baby's 80% development in the scans. Whenever I drank less water, I could feel something stuck into my intestines and it was hard to even breath. Later, the doctor advised me to do brisk walking and squads. It was the 9th month. Almost at its end, when the doctor told me that I have to go through C-section. I couldn't speak for moments as I had never thought about it and I was not at all prepared for it.

I started crying, my husband told me that it will affect me and my baby, so stay calm and make the decision. Even if I did not want to, I had to say "Yes." And I planned to go through the procedure after 2 days on 19th June, 2017.

Now was the time when I was both excited and nervous. They took me to the operation theatre. Even at that moment, I was not ready to go through this. And while taking anaesthesia, I was shivering. Doctor had to divert my attention to make me feel normal. After they gave me anaesthesia I couldn't feel anything. Literally, nothing! My lower body part had become numb and so was I.

When the procedure started, all I was thinking was about the baby. Would it be a baby boy or a baby girl? I was happy to have any of these. It was my first baby. And I was dying to hold it in my hand and to see it. Amid all this, I heard a cry. I wanted to jump and remove the blind fold. But I couldn't.

My doctor told me, "It's a boy!".

I screamed in joy "Alhamdulillah! Can I see him?"

"Yes", they said, for a moment they removed the blind fold and I could see "my baby". He was tiny and the most beautiful person I ever saw.

This happened for a few seconds. They took him out. I couldn't even hold him. I wanted to hug him, to kiss him. But I couldn't. I didn't know when I would either. So I was just thinking about him. I was taken out of the OT and shifted to the normal ward. All my family members came one by one, congratulating me for the new blessing of my life. Still, I could not feel my legs or stomach. Later, they gave my baby to me. Now, when the time came to hold him, I was scared to take him in my arms, all these thoughts were running on my mind; if I could hold him properly or not. What if he starts crying and what if, God forbid, he slips from my hands. He was very fragile and too cute to handle. I took him. I hugged him. I rubbed my cheeks to his. My nose to his nose. And he kept his fingers on my cheeks. I didn't want to let him go. But they said he should be kept under observation for three days. So this separation for a temporary period of time was bound to happen.

It was the best and most memorable day of my life. To hold your baby in your arms, to have this great blessing from Almighty is a dream come true. Later that day, when the effect of anaesthesia was getting over, I could feel severe pain in my abdomen. The stitches (the eternal marks on my body) I got while bringing this new life to the world, were very painful. The pain was unbearable. I screamed. Immediately they gave me painkillers (via injection). I felt some relief. Some respite at last. And this continued after every 6 to 8 hrs. I don't know how many injections I took. By God's grace, all this came to an end after 5 days of the delivery.

This was the time to celebrate. We, with our tiny new family member, came back home. Those scars and the pain I endured while going through this phase of my life is embedded in my memory. And I get scared whenever I recall those moments. But, when I look at my child and when I play and laugh with him, I forget everything I have suffered. After Almighty, I find my ultimate happiness and peace by his presence in my life. And that's enough for me to live my life. As they say,

"Children reinvent your life for you"

*****

"Motherhood is the hood that protects children from the creases of life"

~Ronak Shah

Indelible Impressions

~Nusrat Balur

It was a day of "Team Get-Together". After a long time, I was super excited to meet my colleagues and talk many things.

First Trimester: 26th October

I finally reached the venue and was happy to meet them all. There were varieties of foods served to us. From pizzas to burgers and juices to ice-creams, there was everything for an ideal brunch. Something struck me when I took a deep bite into the pizza - A feeling of 'Nausea'! Yes, I felt something unusual. Ignoring the thought, I moved on to relish some desserts and somehow managed to eat comparatively less. On reaching home, I repeatedly thought about it – Why was I feeling like that? Why is this discomfort? It was late night and my husband walked out to buy some medicines. I followed him right behind asking if I too could accompany him to the store. While he was busy paying out the bills for the medicines, I silently whispered in his ear: "Can we buy a kit?"

Hearing this, he burst into laughter and asked, "Have you gone mad?" as this was unexpected.

I replied, "Just for my satisfaction."

That whole night, I was excited as well as impatient waiting for the dawn to arrive and I could check what I was badly waiting for. It was 5 AM and I suddenly woke up, I remembered I had to test myself. I rushed with so much eagerness and positive belief that the test would turn negative for sure. My eyes were fixed at the little instrument – one line turned pink and I

assured myself – 'Yes, this had to come', wait for one more. In no time, the other line turned pink! I could not believe what I had just seen. Yes! I am pregnant! I didn't know how to react – be happy or sad? I ran and woke my husband up who was in deep sleep and told him – "See this." He woke up rubbing his eyes and looked at the kit in the little light falling on the kit in the dark room and asked,
"What is it?"

I promptly replied, "There's another addition to our family!"

It was a moment of joy, a moment of thankfulness, a moment of feeling truly blessed. All the time I wondered, how did this happen under so much of mental stress and later thought to myself that it was a pure blessing coming our way from the Almighty.

Second Trimester: 22nd December

It was a day of happiness; happiness that I could finally take some time out for a cousin's wedding at my native. The train was to depart at 6 AM sharp and we proceeded from home at 5.15 AM. Around 20 kms to be covered in 45 mins to reach the railway station! As we boarded an auto and started moving with the clock ticking faster and faster, we hardly had time to think about other things. We reached halfway and the driver stopped to fill fuel, it was quarter to 6 AM and we were still halfway! Upon our request, the driver rode at 60 kms/hour and all the way, I had to stand up and sit down every time there was a speed breaker. This continued for the rest of the journey and we finally reached the station, there was just 2 mins left for the train to depart. My husband planned to take the luggage while I had to carry my three-year-old son in my arms and my little one in my womb. I had no choice but to summon up all my courage and run as fast as I could in my current condition. Due to my sit-stand action in the auto my legs were almost stiff, and I could hardly lift them up once I got down at the station. I saw the train a few meters away and I thought to myself, "Just try putting your foot forward as fast as you can. There is nothing else to stop you once you board the train." With this thought I managed to run towards the train. With every step my heart started beating faster than ever and my lungs started needing more and more air. I finally boarded the train and almost immediately the train started moving, I managed to escape any untoward incident with pure grace of Almighty.

Third Trimester: 24th March

Sundays are generally said to be the day of enjoyment, a day to rest. But, for me, this Sunday was a day to remember not because of its good memories, it was because of the immense pain I underwent. I was in a gathering and suddenly there was a shooting pain in my left ankle. I took out my pain relief ointment and applied it generously hoping for the pain to reduce but NO, it started increasing and radiated towards my entire foot. I managed to walk away from the crowd to rest for a while sitting on a staircase, but the pain seemed to increase exponentially. I had a recollection of having twisted my ankle earlier in the morning and expected to face some discomfort but never thought that it would reach to this level. I rang up my husband and he somehow managed to take me on his bike and carried me up all the way to his friend's house in the first floor which was just two buildings away. I sat there crying in pain while the ice packs could hardly help. Finally took a paracetamol to get some relief. Later visited a nearby doctor who advised to avoid any kind of oral medicines and tied a bandage around my feet which eased the pain.

7th June

With all the memories of the previous day's festival on my mind, I headed to the clinic for a checkup. My gynaecologist asked, "How many movements till now?" I paused for a moment and thought, was there really any movement since a while? My mind answered NO, there wasn't! I panicked and my doctor advised not to take a risk, to which I finally decided not to wait any further. It was 5.50 PM when I was taken in and within few minutes, I heard my little one's first cry and the doctor announced, "It's a Baby Girl!!". My happiness had no bounds as I took a glance at my little baby thanking the Almighty every moment for having given us such a beautiful blessing.

This was my journey of pregnancy- A journey with memories of ups and downs, with happiness and sadness and a final moment of ecstasy which made me forget all the pain I went through during this journey.

*****

"Thousands of crowns would also fall short for the one who carries paradise under her feet"

~Ramsha Jawaid

Seedling Of Desert

~*Sandhya*

housands of injections, no idea how many tests, no idea how many medicines.I had completely forgotten myself in the affair of all these in the last 5 years. I was tired of visiting doctors. My sister-in-law then told me about an ayurvedic doctor who specializes in cases like mine. I was out of hopes, but for her sake I decided to go Haridwar to consult the doctor.

After 2 months, I revisited the doctor for some tests. There, the doctor asked me about the last date of my periods and all of sudden I was taken back as I missed my periods. Doctor asked me to take the pregnancy test. I was nervous. I went to the washroom and took the test. I was not strong enough to see the results and handed it to the doctor and didn't even look at it once. I have been through this situation many times and wouldn't have been able to take denial once again. I was nervous and pressing my hands. It was when the doctor said that I was "Pregnant". There were tears in my eyes after listening the news for which I have been waiting for so long. He showed me the test kit which was showing positive results. I was on cloud nine after hearing the news. I called my husband Dinesh to tell him that we were pregnant. We both were eagerly waiting for the news to arrive and it did.

In the first trimester, we decided not to tell anyone about my pregnancy as we were scared from our past 2 experiences. I wanted to scream at the top of my voice and tell everyone about the good news, but was scared at the same time. My first trimester was a mixture of all these emotions.

From the beginning of second trimester, I started feeling irritated, yet my husband took care of me in a great way. It was time for check-up. We went to Haridwar for that. Sonography was to be done. For the first time we felt and heard the heart beat of our baby. I was having good a health except for the blood pressure. Doctor asked me to take care of the same.

Finally, it was the time to share the good news with the family. No one took it seriously when we told them about my pregnancy, but when we showed them the reports they were all happy for us. Our parents, siblings all were there with us in our happy news.

Dehradun to Haridwar was quite a travel. Hence, we decided that I must stay with Dinesh's brother and sister-in-law in Haridwar. Dinesh used to visit me every now and then

One day, while I was chit-chatting with my sister-in-law, I felt the first movement of our baby. I was eager to tell Dinesh about this and also wished that he was there with me.

I was 5 and half months pregnant when my younger sister got engaged. I went to Dehradun for the occasion and was very happy by being with the family. Hence, completed my second trimester.

After few days, I felt first kick of my baby. I asked Dinesh to come and stay with me and our baby for sometime. We had been waiting for so long to feel these kicks and movements. I used to miss my family. We used to talk on calls but nothing can replace the touch of another. I was happy there too with my brother-in-law and his wife, but I missed my family. It had bad impact on me. My blood pressure started rising slowly but gradually. Doctor gave me medicines for that and asked me to take care.

It was the end of 7th month when I was not well and had to be admitted to Jolly Grant Hospital.

For some days, I was kept under observation. We were scared and various negative thoughts came in our minds. These were one of the reasons that my blood pressure was rising.

The nurse, who took care of me in the hospital, was the one to whom I shared everything about my pregnancy. She guided me and told me that all the negative thoughts were having negative impacts on my baby.

It was the 8th of August, around 10 a.m. when I was rushed to operation theatre. It was not the first time. But for the first 2 times, I was given anaesthesia but this time I wasn't. I was scared. They gave me anaesthesia in operation theatre. I woke up at 4p.m. When I gained consciousness I saw faces of all my loved ones, they were scared and nervous, I looked around the room and my baby was missing. By this time, I was sure that something went wrong and I have lost my baby.

When I asked they told me that the baby was in incubator. I thought they were lying to me and would tell me the truth only when I would be a bit stable. But it didn't happen. I started fainting, it was then when I heard a voice,"take care of the mother, the baby is to be fed now." I got all my energy back when I heard "mother of the baby". I was finally relieved and had gained my stability and went to see my baby. It was a boy, my baby boy. I was directed that my name is written on the cradle of my baby.

When I saw his face, I was smiling with tears rolling down my eyes. I was nervous while touching the baby. Finally, when I hugged my boy I felt that my world has come to life.

I wasn't able to complete my third trimester yet I was able to hold my world in my arms.

*****

"The heart and soul of a mother is masterpiece that fulfils every single desire of a dynasty"

~Bhawar Kumawat

ABOUT
FAMIAN PUBLISHERS

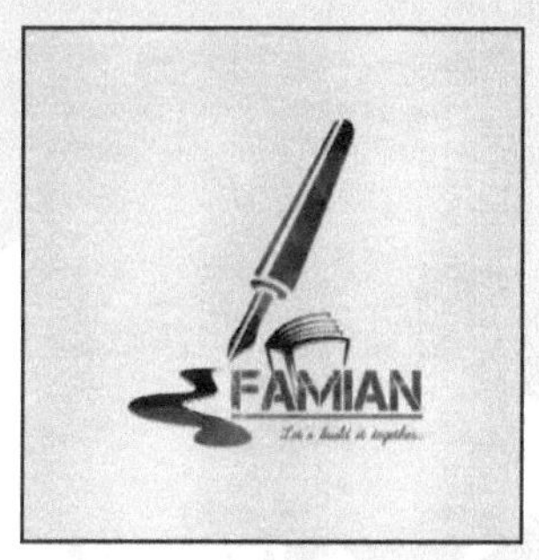

FAMIAN is an official online writing as well as publishing firm. Along with its platform brands- **Heart's Database** and **Writer's Paradise**, it is the sky for Young Writers where they can unfurl their wings and can fly in their own arena. It is a platform to boost up the power of imagination of every author which they actually had never imagined.

FAMIAN is not just a platform and firm to express but also a station for encouragement, enthusiasm and improvement.

Today, where every digital-social interaction counts, it tries to do its best by making every interaction more inspirational. The work is online based as of now. Famian is registered as a Government recognized startup on 31st May 2019, but their work is into consideration since 2018 through the associative platforms -

Heart's Database and Writer's Paradise.

❖ Heart's Database – Since 2017

❖ Writer's Paradise - Since 2018

You can reach FAMIAN at:

famian.onl9@gmail.com

@famian.31

https://www.facebook.com/famian.31/

ABOUT WOMANIYA APP

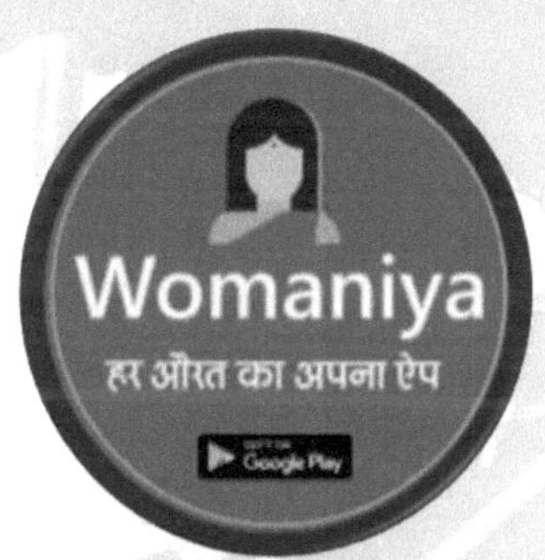

Launch date: 22nd June 2018

Womaniya is a platform for pregnant women to get verified information and support from doctors/experts.
Download the app from below given link :
http://bit.do/fqZGU

Founder : Siddharth Kothari

Contact :
Cell :9930787798
Email id :siddharth@womaniya.co

OUR
INSTITUTE SPONSORS

TECHNO KAKSHA

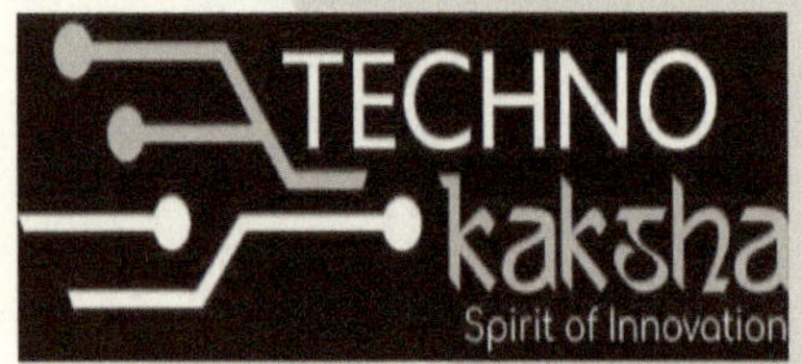

Address:
K.H. No. 24, Plot No. 6,
IGNOU, Main Road,
Saidulajab, New Delhi

Techno Kaksha "Spirit Of Innovation" is an institute of computer software, Hardware Networking and Multimedia, Animation established in 2016.

As a committed and dedicated organization, it is their goal to maintain a learner focus in providing accessible and quality education to directly prepare our students for further study or careers in the Information and Technology, live performance in many fields, audio/visual, working on machinery, event performances, working on live graphics media, working on 3D and media production, working on film industry, photography and Business Growth and some other specialized courses.

Institute feels the underlying concepts of new technology and tools along with reasonable skills be delivered to the students before they go out in the industry of information technology covering software, hardware & live entertainer.

<u>Contact:</u>

Instagram: @technokaksha
Email Id: info@technokaksha.com

Website: http://www.technokaksha.com/
Phone: (011)41724354
　　　　(+91) 8447991962

RAIEDUCOM INSTITUTE OF INFORMATION TECHNOLOGY (RIIT)

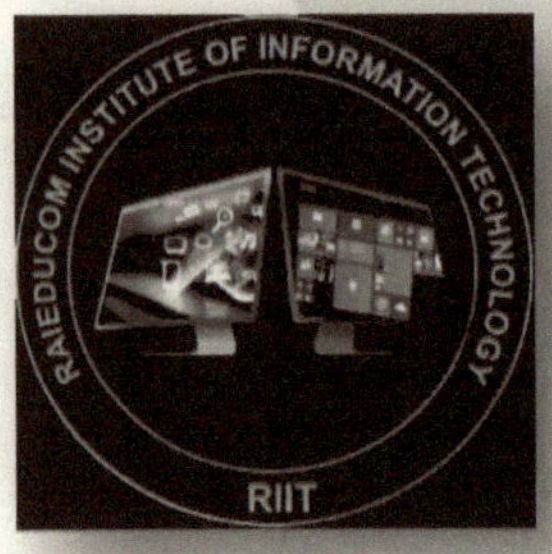

Address:
Kh. no. 24, Plot No. 6, First Floor Saidulajaib Village, IGNOU Main Rd, Saket, New Delhi, Delhi 110030

RIIT works in Hardware and Networking, it's specialties are Software Engineer, Multimedia, Cloud Computing, Digital Marketing etc. It was established in 2017 at New Delhi. RIIT provides training in various sectors. If you want to learn more about then contact and follow in the given below link.

<u>Contact:</u>

Instagram: https://instagram.com/riit_edu?igshid=glo3i94lgfpc

Email ID: eduriit@gmail.com

Cell : 9599157616 || 9871587191

OUR
LITERARY SPONSORS

B.S.R A.S.A Diary 786

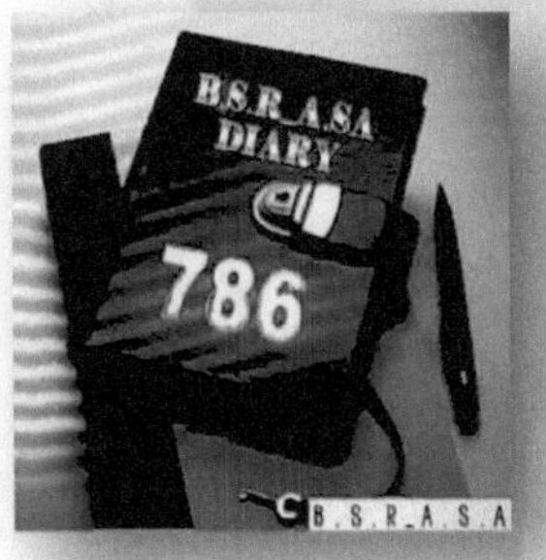

Yourquote Handle:
@bsr_asa_diary_786

Started on :
30th July, 2018

B.S.R A.S.A Diary 786 is a page on YourQuote app which takes you towards the Beautiful journey of Writing, where you can read heart touching poetries, shayaris, quotes and other forms of writings. This page is all about the experience of life and true feelings. Common language has been used in all the writings, so that the readers can be made aware of the purpose of writing. One can feel some hidden feelings and emotions by visiting this page.

Do check and follow this page for amazing experience.

Instagram : @b.s.r_a.s.a_diary_786
Visit the page via this link :
https://www.yourquote.in/bsr_asa_diary_786

Contact:
Email Id : sadafrehan356@gmail.com

ALFAAZ -E -AZMI

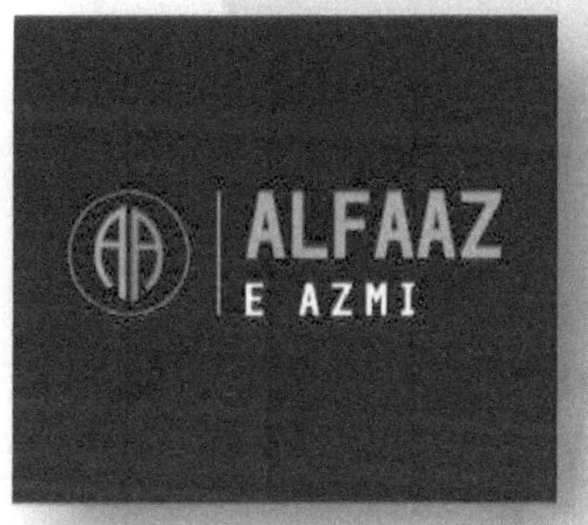

Instagram Handle:
@alfaaz_e_azmi

Started on :
22nd July, 2017

Alfaaz E Azmi is an Instagram Page which is started in 22nd July 2017. The Page is started just to save the voice of creator's heart at place where it is safe and accessible whenever want and later it changes into the voice of so many Hearts.The page have a wonderful collection of Shayeri and Quotes related to real life, love, and other relationships.

Do a visit at least once @alfaaz_e_azmi and don't forget to give an honest reviews on the writings and if you find that the writings related to you then connect with the page.

You can easily follow the page by using the link,

https://instagram.com/alfaaz_e_azmi?igshid=mxuc8okf7prs

IMMATURED WRITINGS

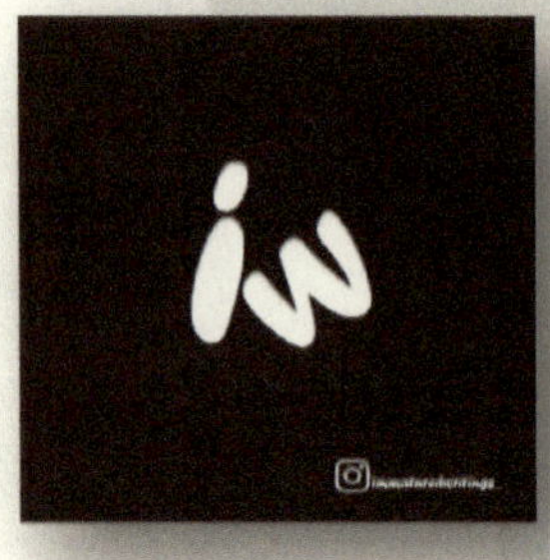

Instagram handle :
@immaturedwritings

Started On :
13th May,2019

Immatured Writings is basically initiated by an immatured boy streaking out his emotions through words. Working on every type of writeup such as quote, shayri, poems, short-stories, microtale, etc . Hindi-english both languages are in use here . Even some regional likes haryanvi, garhwali, gujarati are also appreciated . It's not about promoting any other person . That whole page belongs to one person . All write-ups are originally written . It works on just one motto : 'Immatured streaks and deals with all of us' . Visit for some good work .

<u>Contact Info:</u>

Email id : immaturedwritings@gmail.com
WhatsApp: 9911169729
Instagram: @immaturedwritings
Twitter: @solitaryshayar

OUR
CORPORATE SPONSORS

PRO RICH

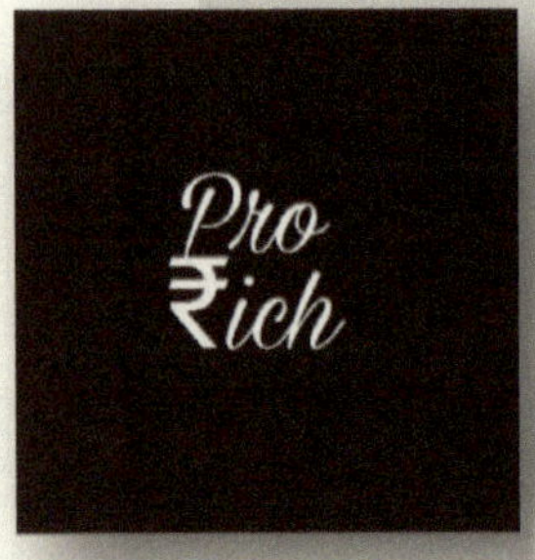

Instagram Handle:
@manishbhatia

Address:
Mumbai,Maharashtra

Pro Rich is a financial advising facility by Manish Bhatia who is a personal financial advisor. He specializes in mutual funds and insurances. You want to grow your money but don't know where to invest?

Call and get all your questions answered free of cost.

You can Visit this link too,
Facebook : https://www.facebook.com/manishbhatia69/

Contact :
Cell : 9820191569
Email id : mbhatialoans@gmail.com

Pk Metals

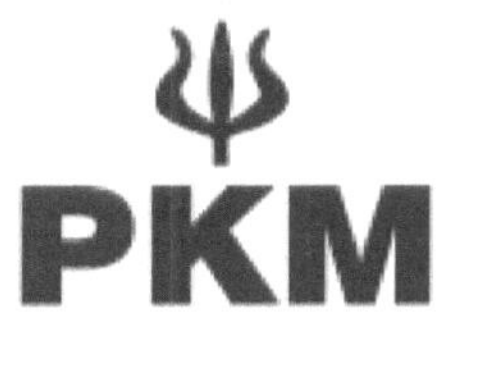

Address:
No. 38, vengu chetty st Park
town ,Chennai,
Tamil Nadu -600003

P K Metals is a leading brand in field of stainless steel business. Doing a wholesale business in Tamil Nadu to leading shops and companies from past 25 years. Dealing in different kinds of finished goods and gift articles.

For more details, contact,
Email id : pkmetalchennai@gmail.com

Cell : 1)044-25331710
       2)9710359167.

BRANDIT

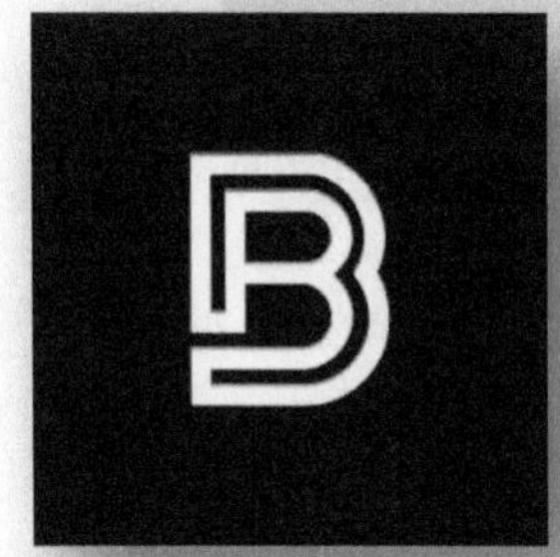

Instagram Handle:
@branditfast

Brandit is an organisation of graphic designers providing all types of graphic design services. It has very reasonable prices and exceptional quality of work. Contact brandit on Instagram.

Get in touch and connect on instagram via below given link:

https://instagram.com/branditfast?igshid=mckxljmk7xuu

CHARISMATIC WORLD

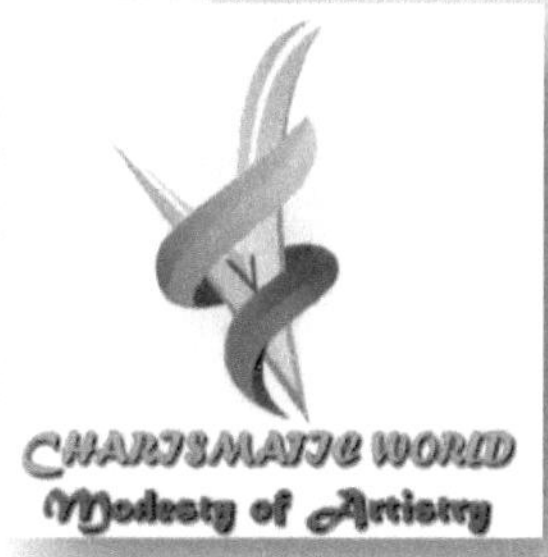

Instagram Handle:
@charismaticworld_

Started On:
28th February, 2019

Charismatic World -"Modesty of Artistry" was established in 2019. She has a collection of different types of artists, also searched latest collections and give platform to new comer artists. Showcase artist collections in one platform. The hub was born out of a vision to build an institution dedicated to Indian art, and the need for a professional platform to connect artists with art lovers. Modesty of Artistry has immense and epic collections of images and music tracks, are the classic choice for everyone to create future dream film. All the photos have a feel of being professionally photographed. She has always welcomed for those artist who wants to collaborate.

Get in touch with the below details:

Email Id: charismaticworld@gmail.com

Tech60's

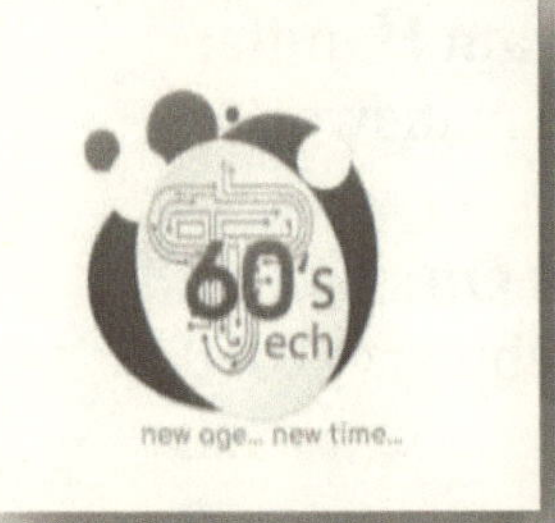

Address:
K.H. No. 24, Plot No. 6,
IGNOU, Main Road,
Saidulajab, New Delhi

Tech 60's is a provided services for New time of New Age generations and launched curator hub and fit 60's for elder people. Tech 60's provide services to senior citizens who can't move anywhere from home services covering Tech Mob, Tech Computing, Fit 60's, Curator Hub, Performing Arts and much more. Their aim is to get a personal assistance at your place for fitness and elder care.

Get in touch and stay connected with Tech 60's .

Contact:

Instagram: @tech60.s
Cell : (+91) 8447991962

OZONE FLORA

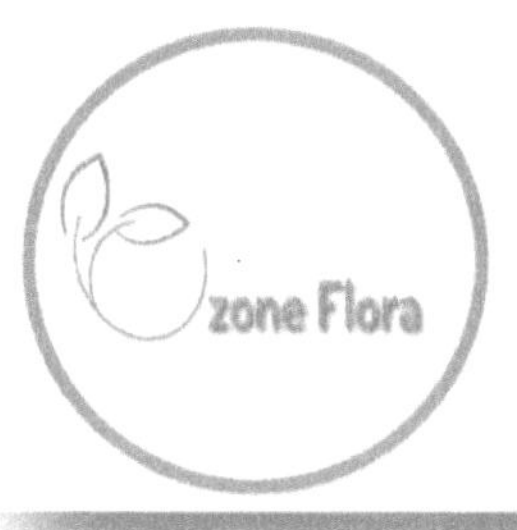

Instagram Handle:
@ozoneflora.co

Address :
Mumbai,Maharashtra

Ozone Flora integrates urban lifestyle with NATURE and health indoor plants with customized pots and décor which improves air quality. They provide shipping across India and deals mainly with indoor plants and customizable pots.

Follow Ozone Flora on instagram,
https://instagram.com/ozoneflora.co?igshid=1qqc0i34r8nt6

Contact :

Email.id : ozoneflora@gmail.com
Cell : +918329349203

LIGHTS N LENS

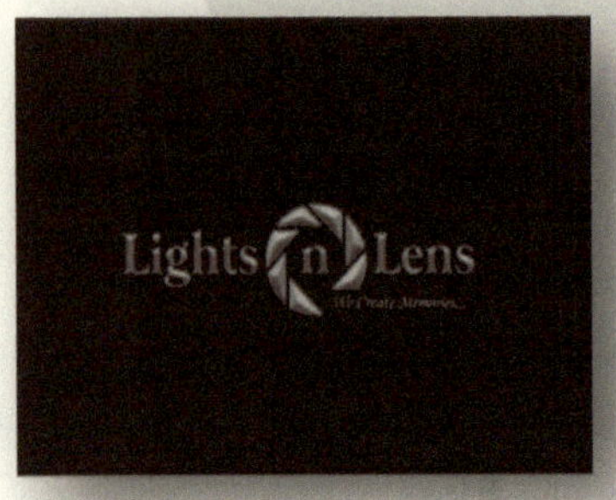

Address:
Survey No. 176/1, Varca
Village, Goa- 403721

Lights n Lens is a contemporary professional photo studio with studios in Mumbai, Lonavala and Goa. Offering contemporary portrait photography services for New born, Wedding, Pre-Wedding, Portfolio, Portrait, Birthday parties, Family, Children, Matrimonial, Corporate events, Fashion, and many more.

Contact :

Cell : 7774847702